Osteopathic Principles

Applied in Mechanics and Treatment

ROBERT JOHNSTON

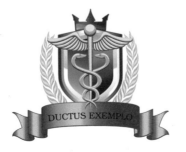

DUCTUS EXEMPLO

WITH ASSISTANCE FROM
DARREN DAVID

ILLUSTRATED BY
JENNIFER HERRING

Osteopathic Principles: Applied in Mechanics and Treatment
Copyright © 2016 CAO Press

Robert D. Johnston
With assistance from Darren David

ISBN 978-0-9949471-1-6

Canadian Academy of Osteopathy Press
The Canadian Academy of Osteopathy
66 Ottawa Street North
Hamilton, Ontario, L8H 3Z1

Formatted and illustrated by Jennifer Herring
Cover & chapter dividers designed by Jennifer Herring
Copyediting & publishing consultation by Dr. Jeffrey Douglas
BSP Communication Consultants, London, Ontario

I would like to thank all those who were instrumental to my education, and those who supported the CAO in its earliest years of development. Most of all, I would like to thank my students for pressing the boundaries of osteopathic principles. Your quest for knowledge inspired mine, and allowed me to understand Still's discovery all the more.

CONTENTS

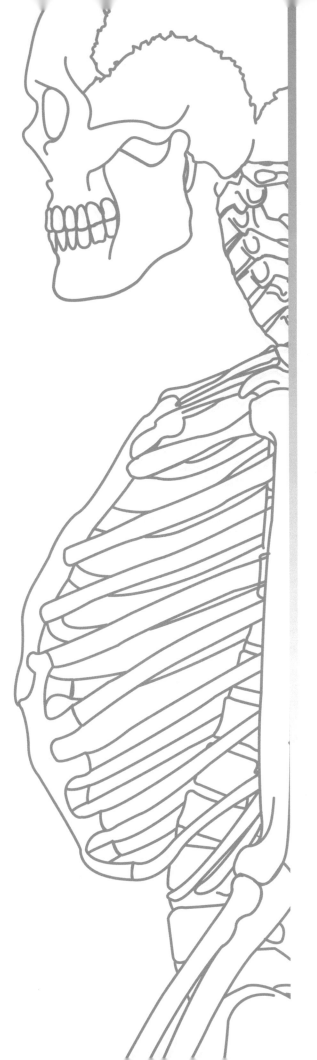

Preface

PREFACE

A Clinical Work

The pages that follow reflect the culmination of a life's work in the practice, education, and promotion of Early American Stillian Osteopathy. To be clear, this book is not a scholarly monograph on osteopathy, but a principles-based book for the practicing clinician. As such, any academic readers searching for quotations, references, and historical timelines from early osteopathic literature are invited to look at the original texts themselves; in this way, the reader can determine how our experiential research is aligned with the founding discoveries that aid in the delivery and effectiveness of treatment. The goal of this project has been to consolidate the common threads of these foundational texts—championed by the works of A. T. Still—and present them in an updated, workable methodology for the modern practitioner. As this is an introduction to osteopathy, the reader should not be looking for definitive answers, or for a comprehensive guide to the application of principles concerning mechanics, diagnosis, and treatment. Rather, this text is meant to plant a seed of knowledge in the budding osteopath.

The truth of the matter is that the current state of osteopathy is fragmented. In presenting this work with our focus on the clinician, we are hoping to forge a united front for osteopathy that does not favour any particular school or approach. Instead, we want to include the best of what each faction has to offer within the greater framework of osteopathic assessment and treatment. If we go back to the basics of practice—to regarding anatomy through our current understanding of physiology—there is little to hold us back from evolving the principles initiated by Still and the early osteopaths. To this end, our desire is for practitioners to bring their voices to the discussion of the osteopathic lesion in ways that advance the science by yielding better results in the treatment room.

We cannot afford to have excessive intellectualism, or ego, dominate the discourse of osteopathic praxis. If we wish to ensure the survival of the profession, the channels of communication need to be opened and extended to all those practicing manual osteopathy around the world. In other words, we need to unite our efforts to reassert our collective position as tangible contributors to improving the quality of life for all people who seek osteopathic treatment. We owe this to the founder of osteopathy, A.T. Still, and to those men and women who faithfully aspired to see his work succeed. By viewing osteopathy through the lens of its origins, we are humble in our approach but unflinching in our proposal, as the founding members would have wanted.

Layout

This book is the collection and integration of much that is good in osteopathy. While compiling this work has been no easy task (as we have also had to sift through the bad), our approach is based on rational inference through clinical application and logical deduction of the anatomy, physiology, and mechanics of the human body, as laid out by A. T. Still, the founder of osteopathic science. We have endeavoured to make this information digestible by those both seasoned and new to osteopathy.

The book is divided into four sections: (1) a philosophical introduction to the Principles of Osteopathy; (2) a discussion on Collective Mechanics; (3) an explanation of Principles in Collective Treatment; and finally, (4) a clinical application with five case studies that serve as examples of how the previous sections come together. These four divisions will help readers navigate the book for studying purposes. By the end, however, it will be apparent that there has been only one topic of conversation throughout: osteopathy. When we are discussing mechanics, we are really talking about treatment; when we are writing about the upper limb, we are really investigating the lower limb; and when we are addressing the philosophical differences that exist in current osteopathy, we are really highlighting the functional anatomy and the physiology involved in the diagnosis and treatment of the osteopathic lesion.

Section I

In the first section of the book, we discuss many of the challenges practitioners of osteopathy face and provide a roadmap to navigate the terrain leading to a promising career in the service of their communities. We also address the fragmented landscape that is osteopathy in order to begin a conversation that brings all those practicing our science to the table so that constructive discussions can take place. Through these necessary dialogues, we can realize an evolution in our practice. To do this, we tackle some difficult topics, including what it means to be Classical, Stillian, or Eclectic osteopaths. For some, this will not be a comfortable component of the book, but if we are to evolve as a profession, it is essential to be open and honest with our assessment of what constitutes osteopathy as defined by the founder. Our goal is to give clarity to practitioners who do not have the time, instruction, or experience to fully understand the philosophies underlying their professional obligations. We end this first section by demonstrating how these philosophical precepts can affect our treatment methods—which begins with palpation. In particular, we approach the barrier model in a more novel way that reflects the three levels of lesioning that should be quantifiable to any and all practitioners.

Section II

In this second part, we delve further into the barrier in relation to the osteopathic lesion, focusing on why or how it materialized. To do this, we comprehensively analyze what we call Collective Mechanics, which is based on a polygonal model of how the body loads and distributes force to promote and maintain health. We begin with the axial frame and then move to the limbs, both lower and upper. In doing this, we schematize many of the findings discussed at the end of Section I, but do so in a way whereby the body can be read osteopathically (instead of merely committing anatomical data to memory). From our perspective, an open approach allows great freedom regarding how practitioners apply treatment to take advantage of the functional anatomy and the body's desire for health. This section is the heart of the book, as it establishes the keystone for our treatment process and extrapolates our philosophical view—a philosophy based only on the principles of osteopathy and our understanding of functional anatomy. Our goal is to corroborate an osteopathic way of thinking about the body that then leads to a more collective approach to treatment.

Section III

Section III augments the key themes of Section II by emphasizing the causative effects that result from our different perspectives on diagnosis, sequencing, and treatment. Here we discuss the principle of correlation, which focuses on a differential diagnosis based on the Collective Mechanics as covered in the previous chapters. We then propose a methodology that is both logical and particular to each practitioner and individual patient. This is neither a routine nor a technique-based approach; instead, it is a way of enacting the principles as deemed necessary by the functional anatomy and the level of maturity and knowledge of the osteopathic practitioner. We then identify the specific qualities and characteristics that result from this carefully thought-out, principles-based approach. Ideally, these elements will assist readers to better understand their goals of working with the body rather than formulaically performing techniques and forcing their will on patients.

Section IV

In the final section, we have compiled some exemplary Case Studies that model classically principled approaches to osteopathic diagnosis and treatment. They are not meant to be definitive in any way. These are attempts to unite theory and praxis, to bring the previous sections to life, and to foster a mindset that will guide practitioners to the most important clinical factor: the thinking osteopathic practitioner is safe, qualified, and effective. Readers should approach this section as a guide to further develop their osteopathic understanding of how the body works, and how osteopaths can facilitate the healing mechanisms inherent in the body. By scrutinizing the anatomy and physiology as the founder intended, we can observe a certain grammar to the body that is reflected in its mechanics, which are dictated by the anatomy. It is from this perspective that we are able to read the corpus and react to our findings by aiding the body, through its structure, to find health.

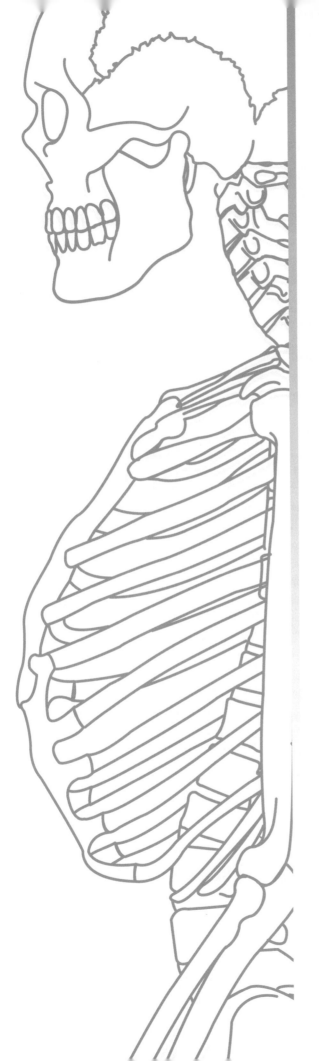

Section I:

A Classical Approach

SECTION I

A Classical Approach

1.1 Engaging the Potential Osteopath

A Challenge at Every Turn

A life in osteopathy is not a simple path. Those who are called to it are individuals who aim to ease the suffering of others with the understanding that their success can only be measured over a lifetime of practice. Those who find success do so by continually improving their knowledge of anatomy and physiology, their ability to assess, and their ability to provide treatment. To this end, this book is in service to devoted practitioners, new or seasoned, who continually seek to inform their minds, to temper their spirits, and to do good work in their communities.

We liken this practice of cultivating the mind to the tending of a garden. To begin a garden, we first must prepare the ground by removing weeds and breaking up the soil. In education this includes breaking bad habits, uprooting incorrect learning, and weeding out unproductive behaviour. Next, we plant a seed, provide it adequate water and sunlight, and hope that it takes root in soil where it can find all the nutrients necessary for growth. This book, like the soil, holds the material necessary for growth within the profession of osteopathy. With the right maintenance, light, and water, that plant begins to thrive—but weeds also find a way in. We must repeat the cultivation process diligently to ensure the environment is conducive to sustained development. This continued practice is something that skilled practitioners know and embrace each and every day, learning from the successes or failures of the past while steadfastly tending to their own garden.

The Need for Contextual Understanding

Even after we become seasoned practitioners, continued education is necessary. Not only is this profession demanding to *first* learn; in order to ultimately master it, a lifetime of self-examination and reflection is required—particularly with respect to the principles set forth by the founder. It is also important to build context for an osteopathic understanding of the anatomy and physiology, which is necessary for every cogent and effective clinician. Such an understanding comes from revisiting the cultural, sociological, and historical knowledge pervading the mindset of Still and the early American osteopaths.

There was certainly wisdom in their approach to developing the science of osteopathy in those early years, which is why they speak so adamantly of *principles*. In these foundational texts we find the progressions of understanding that lead, ultimately, to more intelligent approaches to treatment. The splintering of the science, and the resulting ideological camps that have risen from philosophical differences, made it necessary to look back to these early writers. We need to continue with the tradition they established as a tried-and-true measure for the evolution of osteopathic thought. It is in this vein, therefore, that we frame our approaches to mechanics and treatment. Accordingly, we attempt to distill these early concepts into a workable model that is flexible, particular, and effective, but that remains true to the founders' principles.

We also take care to acknowledge that the early osteopaths had a distinctly early American view of the world that championed a desire for treatment to be rational and independent in its application of the principles. Of course, it is important for practitioners to be able to think for themselves, to come up with better ways to do things, to continually improve on Still's teachings, and to shed new light on how to treat the body. The first osteopathy books were not designed to be streamlined into different subjects as in modern anatomical or physiological textbooks; instead, they were structured to be engaging. From their perspective, if one does not recognize the osteopathic lesions that cause dysfunction, then what good is a knowledge of muscle spindles or an understanding of liver functions? The early osteopaths understood the need to contextualize (and conceptualize) an osteopathic perspective—a perspective grounded in the osteopathic lesion. This context establishes how osteopathy works and so is essential knowledge for the modern practitioner.

No Origin, No Compass for Modern Practitioners

As briefly mentioned, much of the current osteopathic world lacks general consensus on the understanding for the basis of treatment. For some, treatment is about protocol; for others, it is a routine; and for others still, it is about the innumerable techniques to manipulate a joint or tissue (without understanding the osteopathic lesion as governed by the anatomy and physiology behind it). These different approaches to osteopathy have their various strongholds around the globe; they even influence modern practices in the country that founded the profession. While there are many reasons as to how and why this diffusion occurred, the result of these fragmented approaches to our profession has led to a lack of cohesive identity. As long as Still and the early osteopaths are ignored, this ambivalent identity will fester and make it difficult to build our future from our heritage.

By drawing on the traditions established by Still and the early American osteopaths, we offer a firm footing upon which to establish an identity that focuses on aiding the body in its search for health through the best possible avenues. In this way, practitioners can take pride in their science and, in turn, honour the principles as set out by those who founded them. From this position, the science and practice of osteopathy may once again make great strides in our understanding of the human body and how it strives for health. To assume we have already discovered all that the body has to teach is arrogant; there is much more to discover. Let us move forward in our practice with reverence for the human body and a spirit of discovery.

A Context for the Principles

A discussion on the principles themselves without the proper context might also create problems for practitioners. As a principles-based practice, there is much up for interpretation among different schools of osteopathic thought. By itself, a principle means little if it is not understood with respect to treatment. Owing to inexperience with palpation and correct adjustment methods, in the early stages of education the possibility exists of misunderstanding the verbiage used to describe the principles. This is one reason that we return to the original texts and do our best to make sense of how the founders understood the word. We need to contextualize their language to learn *their* approaches to the principles. This is no easy task. Many times, the texts no longer make sense the way they once did: they are written in antiquated diction, and so their metaphors, patients, and scientific language are somewhat enigmatic.

When Still first used the analogy of stagnant swamp water to form an understanding of putrefied blood, his students had concrete experience with the comparison and easily understood the point he was trying to make. Most of today's practitioners have not seen—let alone smelled—stagnant swamp water, and so they are removed from the depth of the analogy's meaning. The same example can be drawn from his use of the term "natural law." While today most of us live in cities, in Still's day, especially where he was teaching, many students were farmers who were intimately connected to the land. They understood natural law because they were part of it; they saw their strong livestock survive, while the weak ones perished. The original references for discussing the principles of osteopathy were simply different from those that we might employ today to feel the same depth and breadth of understanding.

A Resource

It should be clear by now that this book is a bridge from the early American approach to osteopathy to its potentially potent future. As we are transparent in stating our position, our hope is that all other texts that guide practitioners to better ways of engaging our science do the same. That way, other insights gained will not compromise the foundation we seek to fortify and build on, but rather strengthen it to a point where were are able to mature as a profession.

Two Types of Practitioners

Even if we have done our job correctly in establishing a connection from the past to the future, and if the profession matures as it should, there are still risks that reside with one of the two general types of practitioners: those who remain complacent, and those who push forward. While there is little doubt that the methodology we propose will yield results for practitioners, what is in question, however, is how far practitioners will continue to push their understanding of the osteopathic lesion. Will we grow into a profession satisfied in limiting our proficiency to simple strains and sprains? Or will we go back to anatomy and investigate what else is possible in exploring the self-healing and self-regulating capacities of the body? We want to nurture those practitioners who have taken to heart the task of tending to their own garden and cultivating the highest standard for themselves and their profession. Those are the ones who will have the desires and ambitions to discover the full potential of osteopathy as the founder intended.

Technical and Tactical Instruction for Practitioners

This book does its best to mobilize students who have confidence in osteopathy without arrogance within themselves. By laying a groundwork of technical and tactical instruction, we provide the tools for thinking about osteopathy—to understand the *why*—so that students can learn from their mistakes and expand their comprehension. As much as this book instructs, it also challenges readers fixated on their own presuppositions about osteopathy to step outside of their comfort zones, and to do so with eagerness to improve the quality of discourse. For young practitioners, we recommend they be logical and practical in their clinical proficiency and go from easier to more difficult cases, where they will, inadvertently, be introduced to failure. This will either focus or dissuade the student from the growth process. For example, practitioners may be doing well with sciatica, but then fail when they are introduced to a visceral lesion in the same area. The options are simple: either focus on studies and improve technical and tactical approaches for this condition (based on the osteopathic lesion), or pass the patient off to another medical provider. Such a practitioner who passes on their difficulties will see neither the reasoning nor the importance of facilitating an individual's own capacity for healing themselves. By refusing to engage in a complete learning process, the potential of osteopathy suffers.

Aptitude, Character, and Interest

Practitioners, to be receptive to this process, should be chosen not by their academic ability, but by their character, aptitude, and interest, as well as their willingness to have these three attributes tested to make themselves better osteopaths. It is not necessary to have the highest IQ, but rather to be committed to the outcome of care. This means a commitment to the progression of ability derived from a place where success and failure are indispensable components. The journey to excellence is tempered with a tactical and technical approach to the body. It is not about the one case practitioners may or may not have success with; it is about the ability to build awareness of how one conducts themselves in those beliefs. In the end, if readers are open to what we discuss here, they will see that we are talking about the culture of osteopathy. As they engage with the text and its concepts—as they feel connected to its aptitude, character, and interest—hopefully they will choose to become a contributing part of it.

1.2 An Inclusive Vocabulary

This work represents the continuation of an osteopathic discussion from a principles-based perspective. Indeed, our goal is to facilitate discussions around what was once a rich and colourful science, and to inspire readers to become part of an open community that can re-establish itself as a vital constituent of health care. To this end, we are not attempting to write a definitive work that will supersede all others. This is important to clarify as there are many books on osteopathy that try to do just that: seek to be the authoritative word on the subject. All too often, particular schools of thought or communities claim to be the definitive interpretation of osteopathic practice; the reality is that these interpretations are merely one aspect of a multifaceted profession. We recognize how destructive this agonistic approach has been in recent years. If the profession is to survive, we must return to the principles found in each fragment of osteopathy and unite them to build a strong foundation for the future.

When practitioners take a mere fragment of osteopathy and attempt to make it their own—such as offering a course in counter-strain—they do a disservice to the practice from which the principles came. Without a treatment's correct application as determined by the lesion, an artificial representation of osteopathy is the result. Removing the practice from the context of the principles presents a danger to the public, and both practitioners and patients are left with a less than ideal outcome. For us, the question of how to provide quality information for practitioners, as understood within its proper context, is our primary concern. That said, to explain both the art and science of osteopathy is equivalent to attempting to lift the ocean into the air to reveal what's on the seabed below. As we will reiterate throughout this book, *the part cannot be separated from the whole.* To do so results in a series of inconsistencies that negate the totality of osteopathy. Instead, we need to find ways to explain the ocean floor, while leaving the water and all the elements that inhabit it intact. To accomplish this goal, we must rely on ingenuity, dexterity, and flexibility while having confidence in our ability to dive deep into these waters.

From here, we begin a conversation that is free from dogma, ego, and self-indulgence in the hope that others will contribute to the knowledge of osteopathy for both its own sake and the sake of the public we service. Instead of proposing a definitive language on the subject of osteopathy, we offer our understanding of the principles of mechanics and treatment that are best able to restore health. For example, we will discuss quadrants, polygons, and frames, as well as theories of correlation, integration, and balance. They are all part of the same whole. The anatomy does not change. The mechanics do not change. If we are doing our job correctly, our understanding of anatomy and mechanics *will* change so that the early American osteopathic texts reanimate for the modern reader in a logical, productive representation. With a firm understanding of the anatomy, mechanics, and principles for treatment as originally intended, the continued success of osteopathy will be collectively sustained by us all.

1.3 When is Classical not Classical Anymore?

"Classical" as a modifier refers to an idea, principle, or philosophy that came before a significant change in practice. This reference to Classical Osteopathy—the one we present to readers—as its own isolated school of thought is necessary because osteopathy has changed since its inception. It has become either eclectic in its approach or fanatical in its steadfastness. The eclectics (those who borrow from various osteopathic disciplines) will always be around to do what they do. The fanatics (those who attach themselves to one particular name or movement, regardless of who or what that name represents), however, can be dangerous for both patients and the profession. To be clear, simply because the term "Classical" is used by eclectics and fanatics alike, this does not mean it is correctly ascribed. It is important that we always remain critical, logical, and practical in our approach. We must examine what is being presented to us, and be critical of that information by using scientific reasoning. We need to see how the principles withstand empirical, rational tests with an awareness that rationality is not always the most popular position to take.

In modern times, science has contributed more to our knowledge of the body than what was available in Still's time. We should be able to use this current knowledge as part of our diagnostic toolkit to either verify or deny the theories of the past; at the same time, we must be rational enough to change our minds when needed, and to defend the truths that have been revealed and supported through empirical findings. We make this claim because we remember that Still was a free and progressive thinker, one who founded the science of osteopathy on the plain notion of *cause and effect*. He saw that the mechanics of the body had a direct correlation to its health. Because medicine at the time of osteopathy's discovery was not as it is today, we are left with this question: What would Still's thinking be in our modern times? What we know is that fanaticism steeped in the past does not do justice to the classical movement.

We do not wish to marginalize ourselves with bold statements that do not help the profession. Sometimes conventionalism is the best option. Does this mean, then, that we are not Classical if we choose to combine modern and traditional approaches? Of course not. It means that we are Stillian, and that we are principle-based in our approach. Truth is never held by any one individual or school of thought; as practitioners who aspire to be free thinkers, we cannot let any single philosophy dominate our minds. Again, we must be rational in our approach, keep what is useful, seek out the new, and encourage others to do the same. This is how we can keep the profession alive and vibrant.

1.4 Setting the Stage for a Stillian Approach

Defining Our Terms

It should be evident by now that we are quite concerned with Classical Osteopathy as a way of distilling, and then exploring, the potential of the principles laid out by Still and the early osteopaths. For us, the Classical approach should be a progressive one. It should also be clear that we are concerned about how this progress unfolds. This book is not about techniques, however, as it does not attempt to pass off something old as new. Instead, we are providing the impetus for osteopathy to evolve its technical and tactical approach to treatment. We emphasize this point because it makes all the difference in the type of treatment we want to propose. History proves which osteopathic concepts hold merit, and which do not. We consider all of these concepts—regardless of the political biases they may connote—and bring them together to the best of our abilities.

We want to liberate our practice by taking and building on what is useful in a community that wants to do the same. With this reasoned approach, we acknowledge that we do not have to agree on every point proposed within our scope of practice; instead, we should be able to explore the rationale of different positions, and do so with the confidence that each path will aid our collective search for authenticity.

A Methodology through a Lineage of Principles

It is important to have these philosophical discussions to see how context can shape perception. There are important Classical lessons taught in our curriculum, which we will highlight here. In discussing these perspectives, we hope to show how our approach complements each of them, while also demonstrating our own position in the osteopathic landscape—a lineage that spans from the Stillian school of thought to present-day science. We are making extra effort to clarify our approach because, as we will see with the influence of Body Adjustment (BA) and general treatment (GT) (as appropriated by John Wernham), the principles of osteopathy do not always line up with the practice.

Lines of Force, Not Bones

If readers accept the notion that we ultimately serve the lesion, they will come to the conclusion that we must use the tool that is most efficient and effective for that individual lesion. From this perspective, techniques mean nothing; nor do models of adjustment. Let us now explore the *why* of this conundrum.

From a philosophical and historical perspective, we see the influence of Body Adjustment as the provision of a model that first fortifies the mechanical integrity of the body, and then reinforces the physiology of the patient. It acknowledges the body as an integrated whole, but does so by presupposing the degree of dysfunction as reducible to the body's rate of deformation under gravity. By recognizing how the body endures under gravity, we can explore all pathological vectors and thereby eliminate the potential for disease to take root. This type of reductive thinking allows for any practitioner to balance the lines of force that permeate the body to stave off pathologies. This approach strives to reconstitute the entire structure through an integrative and coordinated treatment of the body (a methodology that has great potential).

Integration is achieved through balancing mechanical understanding with knowledge of anatomical structures. The physiological effects of this method are restorative in that they coordinate changes made to the body. This approach can be incredibly useful, especially when practitioners have not uncovered the patient's true lesion pattern, or when strengthening a weakened constitution via general treatment. Early American osteopaths also took this approach to GT; for them and us, however, it was never intended as the final solution. This method differs greatly from Still's original intension: to stimulate the self-healing and self-regulating properties of the body by treating the lesion as the primary focus.

Still relied on this guiding principle—suggesting operators do less rather than more—by finding the key lesion(s) responsible for the dysfunction. To this end, the pervading question to a GT approach can be formulated in the following way: if we are focused solely on balancing lines of force, are we not treating the effect rather than the cause? By raising this query, we can then see the difference between Still's ideas of self-determination and the BA's universal approach to subsume the particularities of human individuation within a common, manageable procedure. This example highlights the importance of holding the ideological perspective of the early osteopaths in our mind's eye as we consider the osteopathic lesion and the best course for aiding the body on its path to health.

Littlejohn and Still

Perhaps the comparison between Still and Wernham is not equitable, since Still and he were not true contemporaries. We do make this comparison, however, because we know that Littlejohn was first introduced to osteopathy by Still. We also know that, although he might not have been his teacher, Littlejohn did live next to the house where Wernham grew up, and that even if he was not taught by the man, Littlejohn certainly would have had some influence on Wernham, colouring his perspective on osteopathy. We also know that Littlejohn's relationship with the Americans was not always an easy one.

Still and Littlejohn differed on many subjects, but for the sake of this discussion we will focus on their approach to treatment. We can say that Still traced osteopathy from the anatomy to the physiology, while Littlejohn did the inverse. Still suggests practitioners pay attention to the anatomy and correct that which is in lesion and let the body heal itself, regardless of whether or not the physiology was exactly understood. While the results were undeniably profound, explaining and justifying these findings to others in the scientific community was not so easy. (For Still, justifying the results to the larger scientific community was unnecessary; there were people to treat, not academic papers to write.) The difficulty in conveying the results was not because Still did not understand the physiology of his time, but because he recognized that the microcosm served the macrocosm. For example, if a rib were returned to its proper place, it would affect the heart in a positive way. Still had tremendous faith in the individual—both in the practitioner to find and correct the lesion, and in the patient to heal and be well again. Still's understanding reflected the early American ideology of self-determination and self-reliance, a philosophy analogizing discovery in the New World.

Not only was this ideology of self-determination difficult to digest for someone like Littlejohn (who was British). Still's dismissal of the academic importance in exploring the physiological side of osteopathy was troubling. It went against Littlejohn's erudite background, where academic research was a foundational pillar in the temple of civilization. As a result, he was quite interested in the understanding of why the heart improved when the rib was returned to its normal position. Still, on the other hand, had little time for this intellectual exercise, seeing it as nothing more than a theoretical construct at best. Still believed he was being honest in acknowledging the limitation to knowing and controlling every physiological variable to health and prosperity. A lifetime could be wasted on such endeavours, only to have them dashed by some future discovery that made little difference to the application of the correction in the clinic room. In defence of Littlejohn, it is possible that he saw research as a way to build up and protect osteopathy for generations to come. He was careful in his pursuit of an approach that balanced the structure of the human body in relation to its correct or incorrect physiological functions. Again, the difference of approach between these two men was obfuscated by the same ideological underpinnings that remain unresolved today.

Searching for a Middle Ground

In many ways, the BA is a step toward a middle ground (albeit one closer to Littlejohn than to Still). With this routine, Wernham focused on the mechanical understanding of integration, coordination, and balance, which regards the structure of the body as a unit and seeks to provide the best chance to improve its overall functions. That said, it was not everything he had to offer, but rather what he felt was pedagogically impactful, that could be utilized by the greatest number of people to get the best average of success. We hope it was not, however, what he would have considered the final solution for osteopathy. Those who see Wernham's contributions as the be-all and end-all of osteopathic treatment can fall into a fanatical fervour at the thought that something else might be possible in osteopathy (much to, we imagine, Wernham's chagrin).

Eclectic Education

The BA is one example of how practitioners have tried to cope with understanding the principles of osteopathy, for we know how vast and all-consuming the practice of this science can be. It requires a great deal of faith to stay on the path navigated by our precursors and see what osteopathy really has to offer; for this, we need time, discipline, and practice. Too often practitioners give up on these basic tenants for success in hopes of finding the silver bullet. The pursuit of catch-all panaceas is dangerous for numerous reasons. First, one's osteopathic garden, so carefully nurtured during the education phase, is left uncultivated. What is true of both British and eclectic osteopathy is that they become ardent at defending their respective positions, even when the principles are not on their side (and their gardens are out of order).

As a consequence of this inflexibility, these practitioners paint themselves into a corner. For example, if they support their cranial model as *the* model, then every subsequent piece of evidence must validate and endorse *their* point of view. This tunnel-vision approach necessitates that everything else—be it muscle energy, Body Adjustment, and so on—cannot be utilized by the practitioner. If another camp champions a visceral model as *the* model, then how are the cranial group and the visceral group supposed to grow together as part of the same profession? It is little wonder that other medical practices give osteopathy little credence. Yet how are we to be taken seriously if we cannot even look at our science objectively and collaboratively? If we place ourselves in an all-or-nothing position within any faction, it is easy to lose face as a rational science both within and outside of our community.

To combat divergence, some have argued that we should return to Still. With this sentiment we largely agree—but we do so with a critical mindset. One of the concerns within British osteopathy is that Littlejohn has become an anointed figurehead; thus, some within the profession have interpreted osteopathy wholly through Littlejohn's understanding of the science. As a result, we get frequent misinterpretations that become compounded and proliferated. Through considering all material from the past, then, we must be mindful when sifting through the various editions in order to identify what is valid and what is purely suppositional. The same approach should be taken with Still's writings. Analyzing his texts with a critical eye is what he would have wanted.

Still was an independent thinker and he persistently encouraged others to be the same way. He believed that explanation must be carried out with a sober mind and a steady hand. We will highlight misinterpretations of Still throughout this book, but one such example that resonates is the myth surrounding his teaching of technique. It is postulated that Still did not teach technique, and that he did not want his students to apply treatment the same way twice. To be clear, Still *did* teach technique—a lot of it. However, it was not presented as an arbitrary effect based on the law of averages; instead, it was based on following the lesion. Still wanted the adjustment to fit the patient, which segues to the second point of contention: he was not asking his students to reinvent the wheel every time they treated a patient. Rather, he asked them to follow the lesion and respond to it as dictated by their palpation, correction, and re-assessment. In this way, the operator never treats the same way twice, and in doing so, every tool or technique used is at the practitioner's disposal. The operator can then customize the treatment for the job at hand, or for the individual, as required.

In looking at these two major influences on the science and practice of osteopathy, we see there is still much work to be done. There are indispensable methods to be found in both the British and eclectic models, methods that should be applied as dictated by the lesion. A GT has the wisdom of integration and coordination until the underlying lesion can be uncovered, or the constitution of the patient can be fortified. The Stillian approach allows us to follow the lesion in a more individuated way. Both have merit, and if we refer back to the dictum that the body is self-healing and self-regulating, and that our job is to work with the body in the least intrusive way to stimulate these mechanisms, we are well on our way to moving osteopathy forward.

The General Treatment: A Lesson in Lever and Fulcrum

If a general treatment (GT) is used as a model in the educational material of osteopathic treatment, the principles of palpation, positioning to correction, and adjustment can be instilled. After learning it, however, practitioners should be encouraged to explore different ways of working with the body in order to expand their osteopathic understanding and the potential to treat in any position with confidence and certainty. Over time, treatments should look nothing like a GT, although it is always at the practitioners' disposal.

When dealing with GT, we are discussing technique and principles as one and the same—direct, indirect, and balance; short and long lever; and fulcrum. Everything else is a variation of these components. To the eclectic mind, this can seem a bit troubling. What about counter-strain? What about facilitated release? The "what abouts" are endless. Our answer is always the same. Everything is a variation on the principles listed above. This GT model provides an integrative way of investigating the body. It allows practitioners to use both the short and long levers as diagnostic and corrective tools. It teaches mechanics. It also establishes a context in which to evolve our understanding of osteopathy. As proficiency increases, practitioners learn to differentiate between varying types of barriers, and then to apply the proper amount of force that facilitates the functional changes to the neurophysiological mechanisms involved with those barriers.

Over time, practitioners will extrapolate from the GT model and begin their assessment of the body at any point, in any position, and come up with a working diagnosis that is logical, effective, and (most important) accurate. At that point, they will no longer need to memorize a routine or a compendium of techniques as their tools will be customized by the practitioner for the individual patient. This progression is desirable because we recognize that osteopathy is, at its highest level, both a science and an art. While the anatomy and physiology do not change, practitioners *do*, particularly if they have had the proper grounding in the principles of mechanics and treatment (which we do our best to outline in the pages to come).

1.5 From Philosophy to Practice

Osteopathy as an Experiential Science

Osteopathy is an experiential science. With proper education and practice, most practitioners find that their knowledge and ability to adjust improves over time. This makes the practice of osteopathy enlightening and rewarding on many levels, but it also makes it difficult for those starting out. This book aims to make that transition easier. Learning the theory and rudiments of osteopathy is difficult enough, so if we are able to expedite clinical understanding, application of methodology, and logical approaches to individualized treatment, so much the better.

Although there are no shortcuts to exploring an entire branch of medical science, there are intelligent ways of introducing the concepts and principles that lend themselves to effective treatment and a long, meaningful career. For those who find themselves frustrated by the learning curve, we suggest forging ahead and experimenting with new techniques. As an experiential science, osteopathy is bombarded with "explanations" of this and that technique, but if a student is not yet experienced in clinical practice, the principles have not penetrated the level of understanding necessary to put them into action. If students feel frustrated, they should be disciplined enough in their study to identify their weaknesses and improve their progress. The more they reflect on their learning, the lesser the gap between the unknown and the known. Self-reflection will better equip students to navigate the terrain of osteopathic practice in a professional and progressive way.

We bring this point to the reader's attention because, for many, prior educational experience has failed to instil the attributes that lead to success. Unfortunately, a Western education system has taught many practitioners that they do not have to be responsible for learning beyond what can be achieved with a test score. This belief does not work for osteopathy. A real understanding of concepts and principles is necessary for real results in the clinic room. Mastery of the discipline does not amount from viewing knowledge as compartmentalized— as practitioners do jump from one topic to the next—but is inclusive, cumulative, and holistic. Indeed, practitioners need all of their faculties, as well as faith in the process of education, to approach abstraction and make it concrete.

Palpating the Barrier

If we accept that osteopathy is an experiential science, then we must first address the most important component of developing sensorial understanding of the body. We are speaking, of course, about palpation. We are not thinking about palpation, however, as it is typically described. We must ask ourselves: what is it we palpate in diagnosis and correction? The answer is, quite simply, the barrier. The barrier is part of the palpatory experience identified by our knowledge of the structure and function of the anatomy; it is either normal or abnormal in the facilitation or restriction of motion.

Conventional explanations of the barrier model involve joint play, where there are anatomical barriers that exist as the limited capacity of a joint to move before injury results. Between these end ranges of movement are physiological barriers, which are based on the soft tissues that aid and protect joints from reaching their anatomical barriers and risking injury. Rarely do we find a joint with perfect symmetry in its full ranges of motion within these end ranges. With repetitive strain, injury, and illness, these become restrictive or pathological barriers, which do not necessarily occur proximal to joint surfaces only. They can affect any range of articulation at any level of tissue in the body. When we palpate and motion test an area of interest in our diagnosis, we are looking at these barriers to determine the best course of treatment. Of course, there is much more that we need to consider when palpating these motion restrictions and asymmetries.

Palpating the Osteopathic Lesion

Although the above information about barriers and palpation would suffice for answering questions on a written test, the information is of little use with complex lesion patterns where subjective and pathophysiological symptoms are at play. Typically, textbooks explain that a lesioned area may be acute or chronic, hot or cold, boggy or dry, tonic or lax, and so on. While these qualities are important in diagnosis, they require a deeper understanding of the total lesion picture. Accordingly, determining the levels of lesioning is a topic we will discuss throughout the book. However, it will suffice to acknowledge that we need to know if a barrier is fully or partially lesioned on the somatic side, the organic side, or both. (As a point of clarification: "somatic" and "organic" are older osteopathic/medical terms for differentiating varying systems in the body. We will go into greater detail on these terms in Section III, but for now, consider that "somatic" or *soma* is musculoskeletal, and "organic" or the *organ field* is visceral and includes its autonomic innervation.) We also need to know if it is a primary lesion or part of a secondary lesion complex. Additionally, we must determine if there is more than one lesion chain at play within the total lesion pattern, and, if this is the case, verify whether it is part of an ascending or descending lesion pattern. Finally, we need to identify the levels of lesioning from a complex chain by noting the degree of lesioning from one field to another (be it somatic or organic).

The Osteopathic Mindset

To truly delineate the barrier model as described above, we need to step back and reframe our approach to reflect the inquisitive osteopathic perspective. As we suggested in our introduction, osteopathy begins and ends with a question. More accurately, osteopathy begins with a simple question, and ends with a *better* question. This scaffolding approach to understanding is human nature and is worth considering in the context of the osteopathic mind. Osteopathy reflects, as its *raison d'être*, human experience in its entirety—from the physiological, to the psychological, to the intellectual and spiritual. Osteopathy interrogates the mysteries of life and death. As we grow as osteopaths, the depth and breadth of our experience deepens, but only if we accept that whatever can be known is allowed to exist above and beyond the knowing self. Never should practitioners feel stagnant in their practice; instead, they should have a drive to explore the body from the moving centre of individual experience. This drive begins with palpation.

In accepting this simple notion, something remarkable happens to practitioners. With the potential to reveal and expound the knowledge of the human condition based on clinical experience, operators are more adept at being present with the patient in ways that are totally appropriate and particular to that individual at that particular moment. From here, the practitioner also gains a greater understanding of what their role is during treatment. It teaches them that treatment is a dialogical exchange of information between the practitioner and the patient, and that this exchange cannot be possible if operators attempt to impose their knowledge and/or will on the patient. To this end, the effective sharing of information between the two parties can only take place if practitioners abandon the desire to control the outcome of treatment, and understand that they can only interact and communicate with a patient's lesion. From there, it is up to patients to respond, and the better we listen to what their bodies say, the better chance we have of giving the body what it needs to communicate.

If this conversation about learning does not take place, it usually leaves students with a romantic but abstract notion of osteopathy. We are not talking in abstraction here; we are speaking about osteopathy as both a science and an art founded on our ability to optimally diagnose and treat patients. This is why we begin with a discussion on palpation and the barrier concept, and then provide a methodology for correctly interpreting the messages the body conveys. We are seeking a clinical, sensible, and reliable way to respond with treatment.

Coming to the Bind

When it comes down to it, the abstract becomes more tangible with our discussion of the osteopathic lesion—in particular, the concepts of *bind* and *ease*. The concept of bind and ease has been an accepted principle in osteopathy; it is often relative to the powers of the operator to palpate and identify the quality of the barrier, and then apply treatment to correct it. But again, apply treatment for what? What does "quality of the barrier" even mean? If we are applying treatment to something, how can we communicate *with* the thing we are palpating? What are we really feeling as we palpate and adjust tissue, whether hard/soft, vascular, neurological, lymphatic, and/or visceral? If it is the bind we are monitoring in diagnosis, what is its fix point as it relates to the corrective method of using a lever and fulcrum in treatment? Are they one in the same? Or is there a better way of thinking about the terminology that can inform how we read the quality of the barrier and deliver treatment?

As we venture through our discussions of Collective Mechanics, we will see how we can begin palpation at the OA joint and apply correct, specific treatment in such a way that helps the body manage heart conditions and/or digestive issues. To achieve this end, we follow the presentation of the body in a rational way—through its functional anatomy—to observe how and why a lesion is expressed as it is. With this new position, we are now able to ask a better question: if the barrier is more than we thought it was, what is its actual limitation?

The Barrier is not the Barrier

The truth is: the barrier is not the barrier at all. The barrier is a result of the communication between systems in the body—namely the blood and the nervous system—because the health of the tissue is determined by the proper regulation of supply. If the passageway from one point in the body to the next is faulty, lesioning will result, expressing itself as a barrier. The barrier, however, is not a tangible *thing* per se. It is not tissue—hard or soft, vascular or visceral, lymphatic or neurological—that needs to be adjusted. It is the space between the structures with which we seek to communicate in order to restore the healing properties of the body. Therefore, since the barrier is not a thing, it is not an object or mechanism that we can do *something* to in a physical sense. The barrier is an expression of dysfunction between structures that we attempt to resolve by reinstating continuity between these structures. By returning continuity to the region, the systems that regulate their proper function can perform their tasks correctly.

Ultimately, when we palpate something and notice a bind, we are then able to think of the causal aspects: how it got there, how long it has been there, and the nature of its qualities. With these insights available to us, we are no longer thinking about the barrier as something to fix, but as part of a process of pathological lesioning that has a history in the body, which is mapped out in how the body copes with the breakdown of pathways of communication. Framed in another way, we focus on the barrier in osteopathy to see what happens *between* structures, not *on* them.

To keep the discussion focused on principles, let us consider structure and function and see if we can, from our new position, explore it further. We can say that healthy, functional tissue is pliable and elastic, that it has better physiology, and, structurally, that it is anatomically sound. But what does this mean in relation to the space we are looking to interact with and re-constitute? In healthy tissue, the space is balanced and reflects a healthy environment where proper neural output, as well as proper fluid dynamics, is provided. Lesioning, then, is the distortion of the space between the shapes that then alters the function of those surfaces. As we diagnose and itemize the various types of lesioning (somatic and organic), we can apply a rational approach to each and every treatment without imposing ourselves on, or over-treating, the body. This practice begins with an awareness of how we understand lesion patterns in conjunction with barriers, the confluence of which will be discussed below.

Barriers and the Fully Lesioned Spine

Before we delve wholly into the topic, it is important to reiterate that a lesion is a breakdown in pathways. The barrier, acute or chronic, is a result of a lesion somewhere in the body, which reveals itself because of the disturbance of the delivery of blood and neurology. The more complete the neural expression in the soft tissue, the more lesioned the body. If the neurology is fully engaged on both the dorsal and ventral (somatic and organic) side, we say it is fully lesioned. As the deep and superficial structures have the same innervation, it does not necessarily matter from where the lesion originates—either a viscerosomatic or somato-visceral reflex—since the nervous system will attempt to conceal or contain the lesion (which is why we use palpation and test motion during the osteopathic diagnosis). In this way, the blood, with all of its nitrifying qualities, will be compromised. The longer the lesion has been in existence, the less quality and quantity of motion is found in the affected area(s). The result is the subjective sensation of pain in that area and/or a pathological change to the physiology.

Levels of the Osteopathic Lesion

To demonstrate the aetiology of a fully lesioned spine—an area where there is a change to both the somatic and organic reflex loop—let us provide an example. The purpose of osteopathic treatment is to bring back stability, coordination, and integration of the body so as to enable the self-healing and self-regulating mechanics that already exist internally. When practitioners position patients to open the superior thoracic aperture, for instance, what are they feeling? There are many things that their palpation can sense as they sink into the tissues (from superficial to deep), one of them being the compression of fluids. As the fluid capillaries fill, they push back against the operator's hands; that region is a dynamic interspace where the barrier tells a story about the nature of the arterial supply and the venous and lymphatic return. With hands in place to monitor the fluid's dynamics, they are able to detect the nature of the fascia, the muscular tone, the bony ring that surrounds the aperture, the position of the clavicles, and much more—all of which explicate the nature of the lesion, and guide the body toward the path to health once the lesion is removed.

This is why the barrier is not a concrete thing that we palpate, but rather a medium through which we read, interpret, and react. Palpating is a hermeneutical (interpretational) act; it provides opportunities to sense something different every time we position our hands on a patient, and it is that difference that leads the operator to better questions. (Is there a little or a lot of fluid? Is it hot or cold? Do we need to pump fluid in or out of the area? What happens to the tissue after we make a change? If a lesion is still there, do we then look up and down the chain? Do we look to the limbs? To the hard or soft tissue? To the neurology or to the viscera?) Treatment, from this perspective, is always dynamic. It is based on our palpation of the barrier, our inquiries, and the hermeneutical act of interpreting what the lesion has inscribed on the body. With these tools, practitioners are able to adapt their approach according to their interactions with the tissues of the body, and respond with differential diagnostic methods. Details on this methodology will be discussed further in Section III.

Types of Lesions

Thus far, we have introduced a method of using palpation to develop a working diagnosis of the type and depth of lesioning, the purpose being to better interpret each patient's expression of the osteopathic lesion and lesion pattern. These expressions can range from partially lesioned to fully lesioned, and can be categorized into three areas: *singular lesions*, *chain lesions*, and *complex chain lesions*. We make these distinctions because the pathways to both health and disease are directed by the intensity of each of these three potential abnormalities.

As we map out the lesion pattern based on our palpation, we are able to observe each of these variances in our diagnosis, which then directs our course of treatment. With this in mind, let us explore each of these concepts in greater detail.

Pathways to Health and Disease

A singular lesion manifests as a single pathology. For instance, we note a change to the erector mass along the spine between D5-9, which indicates a possible alteration to the visceral reflex of the upper portion of the digestive system. As we palpate over the ventral abdominal cavity, we are able to confirm this by detecting lesioning over the liver and gallbladder. If there is proximal lesioning in the musculature, common sense dictates that there would also be irritation to the hepatic portal circulation, which would affect the intrinsic neurology of the gastric gland that, if left untreated, could lead to a chain lesion where the pathway between one organ and the next is compromised. In the early stages of the pathology, the lesion is first expressed in the liver, but if left untreated, it could have a chain effect on another gastric organ, such as the stomach.

If we had this hypothetical patient come to us with the expression of this type of chain lesion, where a sluggish liver leads to a gastric issue, the patient might present as having a problem with gastric regulation (such as reflux). In this instance, as the pH from the stomach enters the mucosa of the larynx, its tissue is compromised. Irritation in the throat, compounded with abnormal material coming from a sluggish liver, could result in further lesioning of the esophagus that may eventually propagate any number of related pathologies. All of these lesions are considered a part of the same chain, for they all reside within the gastric system. In this example, we are looking at the logical links between one set of lesioning to another, and piecing our diagnosis together based on our knowledge of functional anatomy. To assume, however, that these "links" represent the extent of the possibilities afforded by the body is short-sighted to say the least.

The same simple gastric lesion in the liver that aggravated the stomach and esophagus could easily have a knock-on effect on any number of other systems outside of the GI system. When there is more than one system in lesion, it is called a *complex chain lesion*. Our goal when reading the body, based on our knowledge of the passages between these systems, is to ascertain the interdependence of systems in confluence with anatomy. For instance, if the secretory glands in the stomach are in lesion, there can also be interrupted signalling at the vagus nerve, which can negatively affect the elimination cycle. As the digestive system becomes sluggish, it holds more of the body's blood, which leads to stagnation of chyme and blood, bloating, and further irritation of the vagus nerve (ultimately raising the sympathetic tone to attempt to move the blood out). Now the autonomics are caught in a pathological sequence that reciprocally charges both systems as they strive for homeostasis, which leads to bouts of constipation followed by bouts of diarrhea. Eventually, the erratic vasomotor tone in the gut, together with the poor nutritive quality of the blood, can have a negative influence on the heart, which is trying to keep pace with the autonomics. The poorer-quality blood then makes its way through the lungs, which then hinders a clean exchange of gases as the blood becomes oxygenated for redistribution throughout the body. Reflexivity along the erector mass of the spine might then become compromised, and we might note lesioning in the upper cervical and upper dorsal regions, as well as in the pelvic region, in conjunction with what we originally found at D5-9.

The examples of lesioning described above are rudimentary vignettes of simple, chain, and complex chain lesions, and are offered as a way of introducing better palpation and diagnostic strategies. Within each of these examples, there are a myriad of mechanical nuances throughout the entire body that could be influencing the type of lesions and how they manifest. As we work our way to the mechanical and treatment portions of this book, we will revisit these concepts in the context of developing a more accurate osteopathic diagnosis.

It Is All about Perspective

Much of the value of osteopathy comes from its approach to the lesion. The greater vantage point practitioners have, the more they are able to ask better questions and, from those questions, determine the pathology and degree of lesioning in the clinic room. This knowledge is essential as it is possible to have two very different patients with different constitutions, vitalities, and life habits who nevertheless exhibit similar pathologies to the complex chain lesion mentioned earlier.

On the one hand, if we observe athletes with athletic postures, their joints are typically fibrosed with shortened tissues. The intensified fibrosis is caused by a perpetual cycle of injury and healing due to overtraining and performance-based conditioning. From this case, it is possible to read the erector mass and note the same lesioning in the areas described in our above example of complex chain lesions. The pathology, however, might originate from a different point, depending on the nature of the sporting activity. For instance, we might observe lesioned tissue stemming from alterations in the soma in the upper dorsals, which then creates back-pressure in the cardiac tissue. This pressure on the cardiac tissue in turn causes a pooling of blood in areas of the body where blood can typically stagnate—in the stomach, for example—which can then lead to, as before, a sluggish digestive system, which can furthermore mutate into a liver, esophageal, and/or heart lesion.

On the other hand, if a patient is too flexible and lacking muscular integrity to keep the soma in good function, operators will notice that the blood is too superficial in the body, and is not supplying adequate nutrients to the deeper intrinsic organs. As a result, the chyme moving through the gastrointestinal tract that dumps into the hepatic portal circulation does not provide the best materials for the liver. That degraded quality of blood then circulates to the lungs for combustion, which leads to (as before) a compromised gas exchange. The quality of blood that then circulates through the rest of the body for upkeep is also inadequate. Degraded blood quality has an overall destabilizing effect, which can cause the patient to succumb ever more to their lesion pattern.

In both of these cases, the lesion originated on the somatic side according to each patient's habits, and made its way into similar complex chain lesion patterns. It is important to see these connections, for even though the origin of the lesion might have been different, the pathology was the same. The point to make regarding treatment, however, is that both patients should require and receive a different procedure—based on their constitution, vitality, and engineering of their bodies—for what might be appropriate for one patient could injure the other (and vice versa). This is why we must be vigilant in our approach to the body, administer informed palpation techniques, and know how to adjust our treatment for the patient we *have*, not the patient we think we *should have* based on protocol for gastric or cardiac lesions. So the question becomes: if we are to make a change to facilitate the healing properties of the body, what do we do? The answer is the one thing that all operators have at their disposal: the mechanics as influenced by the anatomy.

Pathophysiology Reflected in the Mechanics

When we palpate the spine over D5-9, we should primarily note the temperature and texture of the skin, as well as the differences in the bind of the soft tissue. (While palpating, bear in mind that deep and superficial tissues have the same innervation and blood supply.) We will subsequently notice that there is a global sidebend over the liver. The proximal diagnosis would analyze the compression over the liver because inconsistencies in blood pressure, due to back pressure of portal blood, indicates possible lesioning in the liver. As a chain lesion, we see that it affects the rate of nutrification from the digestive system to the liver and the rest of the body, leading to any number of toxic events that could be expressed through the excretory channels (elimination, urination, gas exchange with the lungs, and/or through the skin).

Additionally, we will notice that the sidebend affects the adrenal glands, which could further exasperate the blood pressure and impede the autonomics and endocrine systems. Essentially, discord within the liver can have far-reaching effects on the entire nervous system, heat production, and lymphatics. If we look beyond the sidebend at D11/12, observe the position of the upper T-line, and notice a declination in the upper thorax, then we can deduce that the lung is caught against the rib, which will affect blood flow, gas exchange, and lymphatic circulation. This is a complex chain lesion where a patient presents with numbness and tingling in the left hand, high blood pressure, poor skin quality, feelings of sluggishness, urinary infections, and a cough that will not abate. Of course, this is merely one series of expressions of dysfunction, but in following the lesion pattern as we have described it through polygon mechanics, practitioners can see the thread that unifies all of these symptoms of disease. More importantly, practitoners have a methodology for doing something about those symptoms. From a material point of view, operators can see the body as a dynamic unit of function, and ascertain that a barrier reached at D11/12 (or at the shoulder girdle) can generate a working osteopathic diagnosis; from an explicative point of view, they should see restriction as part of a narrative of disharmony in the body, one that is expressed through the breakdown of communication pathways as reflected in the anatomy.

As we test the barriers in and around the sidebend over the liver, we note what is above and below it, looking for compensation (or the lack thereof). If we note a sidebend and rotation to the opposite side in the upper thorax, we now can differentiate between the quality and quantity of motion between the lesions in the lumbar and dorsal spine. Our diagnosis can then be constructed by prioritizing between the areas of greatest restriction to the least. This will give practitioners a sequence by which to treat either *to* or *from* the primary area of restriction.

Of course we can also use different diagnostic tools (such as dermatome or myotome testing) to guide diagnosis, but operators should be aware these tools are only useful if we consider the whole body as a symbiotic unit. The same is true for monitoring a patient's temperature. With respect to the two types of somatovisceral patients discussed earlier, one body part being hot or cold could have different causes and a dissimilar narrative sequence (chain). A part being hot or cold does not tell us much unless we see it as belonging to a lesion pattern, which can be interpreted based on our findings in the mechanics. We must remember that the body is both a dynamic unit of function and a closed system. If something is hot, something else will be cold (and vice versa). The degree of expression as a proximal lesion, a systemic lesion, or a chain lesion is determined by the constitution and vitality of the individual, and by the duration and formation of the lesion complex. Without seeing the body osteopathically, we miss many diagnostic opportunities that allow us to observe how the body is regulating temperature and where the key lesion may reside.

Conclusion

The barrier is not something that we touch, but rather something that responds to touch. That exchange of information happens in the space between the structures. The sophistication of that exchange is measured by the practitioner's ability to understand the language of the body—to have the palpatory lexis to interpret somatic signs and reconstitute the environment in which the tissue may self-heal and self-regulate. To this end, it is the patient's body that teaches the osteopath when the right questions are being asked. This education will happen over time as our abilities deepen with our understanding and experience. With the notion of "experience" in mind, we will now turn to an application of methodology that puts the information presented in this chapter into practice.

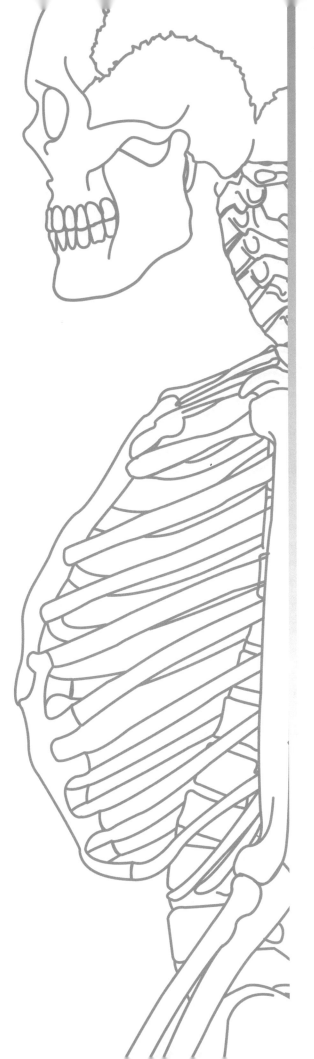

Section II:

Collective Mechanics

SECTION II

Collective Mechanics

2.1 An Argument for Mechanics

As Stillian osteopaths, we know that the primary pathway of communication in the body is the blood stream. We also know that the nervous system plays a central role, but that it has its own blood supply. As a consequence, the health of a nerve—and the organic and somatic tissues it innervates—is determined by the quality of its supply. Palpation of the blood supply is often mediated by the condition of the nerve, but it should always be remembered that the artery reigns supreme. For example, when we palpate and motion test a somatic structure, we are reading the expression of a dysfunctional reflex that is having a direct reciprocal effect on the capillary bed of the muscle. Through treatment, we can have an effect on the GTO/muscle spindle reflexes. The change in that reflex influences both the tonicity of the muscle and the vasomotor tone of the blood vessels that share its innervation. The benefit: overall motor stimuli is lowered throughout the body, allowing the entire corpus to work more efficiently. Our work, therefore, needs to be cautious and concise; the somatic tissue is not our primary concern for its own sake, but rather for the sake of all the tissues and blood supplies it can affect.

Throughout this book, we seek to temper the intensity of ambition within the practitioner. While there are seductive voices that claim to have the master key to unlock shortcuts through the labyrinth of the human body, those voices rely more on argumentative persuasion than on actual reasoning. We want to avoid employing only local treatments that do not attempt to integrate changes made to the body. At the same time, we do not want to disturb every joint in an attempt to coordinate the body and end up overtaxing the nervous system. We also do not want to focus on fluid dynamics, osteopathic centres, visceral models, autonomic distribution charts, and/or subjective complaints alone. All of these tools are important—and they must be available to every practitioner at all times—but they should only be used when needed. Ultimately, we think like engineers and operate like mechanics. This is why we discourage groupthink devoted to one vein of thought, as osteopathy must be inclusive rather than exclusive. We invite those who find themselves developing tunnel vision (often cloaked in the language of "specialization") to liberate themselves by becoming generalists.

Yet we must explain why, within an *introductory* book on osteopathy, we have chosen to focus on mechanics and treatment if we claim to be generalists. To do this, we will examine neurology and fluid dynamics. Upon our initial palpation, we are able to detect differentiation of texture and temperature of the soft tissue before the boney tissue. According to Hilton's Law, we know that if the soft tissue is altered in any way, there is also some degree of hard tissue lesioning because both superficial and deep tissues are inverted by the same neurology. As mentioned above, there are two primary ways of interpreting how such lesioning fits into the disease process.

On the one hand, heat on the surface of the body can mean that blood has moved from deep to superficial in a reflex zone. In this case, the inflamed superficial tissue indicates the organ field beneath it is also inflamed. It also means that another part of the body—from superficial to deep—will be cold and congested. As fluid is non-compressible, it has to move somewhere. If that "somewhere" is prevented from operating as a normal functioning body due to a mechanical lesion, there is now an abnormal displacement of fluid with which a limb or an organ must contend until normal mechanical function can be re-established. In this way, the mechanics that drive the displacement and congestion of fluid, if left untreated, could have a disjunctive physiological effect.

In this instance (as well as in others where the surface tissue is hot), the deep blood has been shunted away from the viscera. Thus, the osteopath's task becomes one of tracking down the mechanical lesion and returning it to its relative normal state. We are not suggesting a tracking method, however, as operators must always follow the lesion pattern. If diagnosis were as simple as *do this for that*, all we would require for treatment is a series of charts, a rudimentary ability to navigate, and some practice at adjusting *this* centre for hot cases, and *that* centre for cold cases, and so on. Success is not that readily attainable, unfortunately, for there are a myriad of factors that could be influencing the dysfunction of the neurovascular system. Ultimately, this is why mechanics are of great importance in this book: it provides a tangible objective for practitioners to use in a clinical setting.

Further Considerations of Mechanics on Fluid Dynamics

If we have an area of congestion, we must map out the vascular pathway that leads to and from that area because, more often than not, if something is cold, then something else will be hot in order to move the blood. Our job as practitioners is to find out why this is occurring. As we will explain, sometimes people have simple lesions, either on the somatic or organic side, which are localized to one area. Other times, there is a chain lesion on either side of the lesion field that includes, on the organic side, paired organs that inhabit a similar space (such as heart and lung) and perform complementary functions. On the somatic side, a chain lesion can either be ascending or descending, moving from one localized area—superficial to deep, or vice versa—to a larger area, limiting the motion of more than one muscle group or more than one joint. Lastly, there can be complex chain lesions that, on the organic side, influence one organ pairing (such as heart and lung affecting liver and stomach, or vice versa). On the somatic side, we begin to lose compensation as we move from one limb, through the axial skeleton, to another limb above or below, left or right. In both cases of organic and somatic, however, there will be a blending of lesions across fields so that an organic lesion is never without a somatic result. The same effect can then be noted extending from the somatic field to the organic because, to reiterate, both fields of lesioning are influenced by the same motor supply. Therefore, we must look to see what pathway between these two fields is in lesion, and is therefore impeding the proper rhythm and continuum of distribution between one area and another. That is where our focus on mechanics becomes indispensable.

For instance, imagine a case where there is a declination of the right shoulder girdle in the upper T-line from the ventral view. From the dorsal view, the girdle will be elevated, and the thorax will show a rotation to the right. The ribs, in this case, will be exhaled ventrally and inhaled dorsally. As we move past the superficial tissues to the deep, we see that a posterior shoulder means that the right lung is also posterior. Over time, a cough develops due to the mechanical compression of that right rotation of the thorax on the plura of the lung. The change in position of the shoulder girdle also affects the position of the arm that further impedes the potential for lung expansion. This leads to fluid congestion on the right, which prevents drainage. To address this congestion, another area of the body gets hot. The blood to the other organ systems is now moving faster to build back pressure to free the obstruction to that right lung. We also have a great deal of back pressure to the heart, which heightens sympathetic tone for its innervation in the upper dorsals and makes it work harder. Owing to this increase of autonomic activity, the intrinsic muscles leading to the neck and head go into spasm, and neck pain results. Where many practitioners make an error is in their structural diagnosis when they observe coolness in the gastric region, which is evidence of back pressure meant to relieve the lesion in the lung.

If we are thinking mechanically, however, we will notice during structural diagnosis that there is a shear between the gastric region, the upper T-line, and the position of the neck. Our proposal, then, is to coordinate these regions through the functional mechanics. Upon motion testing and working through our differential diagnosis, we note that the problem is not entirely a gastric issue. In other words, even though the trophicity and quality of the tissue may be compromised, the primary lesion is found in the twist in the upper T-line and the depression of the ribs on the right side. Should we free that girdle and those ribs, the neurovascular back pressure subsides and all systems normalize.

Addressing the osteopathic centres may have helped in this example, as may have drawing on general treatment or a physiological treatment. Yet each of these approaches are treating the effect, not the cause, and therefore cannot be considered truly osteopathic. All levels and fields of lesioning are important, and while different types of treatment are necessary at different times, they should never be at the expense of following the functional anatomy. We know a pathophysiological state when encountered because a cause or effect shows itself as a distortion of the anatomy. If, then, we base our mechanical model on the functional anatomy, we will always have at our disposal an appropriate diagnosis and treatment plan for each particular patient at that particular time. Having a predilection for one school of thought, or a biased investment in one system over another, can only be a hindrance to seeing the forest from the trees.

2.2 The Mechanical Loop: Anatomy, Physiology, Pathology

It is always important in osteopathy to resist the temptation to compartmentalize our understanding into isolated subject areas. We should not seek out self-contained chapters on anatomy, physiology, and mechanics; instead, we should be more comprehensive in our understanding of the body. We do this in osteopathy because we believe that disease is derived from a malposition of the anatomy. Indeed, the irritation, inflammation, and degradation of tissue that can lead to one pathology stems from discord in the symmetry of the body. These asymmetries affect the position of joint surfaces as well as their mobility and motility; the result is that physiology transforms into pathology. These pathological lesions are not typically isolated to one area. Their lines of force also affect associated structures, proximally and distally, that can be palpated and tested according to the functional anatomy. Functional anatomy can be referenced back to an understanding of the mechanics, which enables communication with each other and with our patients.

The main objective of the present discussion is to provide a way of finding, at the same time, the source of disease and the source for health. We describe this understanding as a loop with mechanics at its centre. The loop sequence progresses from the malposition of the anatomy, to the malposition of the physiology, to the pathology, and back to the malposition of the anatomy. We know if there is a perversion in the anatomy, the mechanical will not function correctly. Physiologically, the sympathetics lead to either a vasodilation or constriction of tissues. This is significant because the body is a closed system; therefore, the autonomics function so that stimulating vasodilation in one area means stimulating vasoconstriction in another. In altered anatomy, both ends of those reflexes are affected. If left untreated, the homeostatic balance between these reflexes will lead to a pathology stemming from the malposition of a joint.

In observing the body collectively through a discussion of how joints and anatomical transition points correlate, we can schematize the body osteopathically. We see how the body attempts to find and maintain health with different patterns of compensation in response to varying types of somatic stresses (such as the malposition of the joint). Without this perspective, it is easy to forget about the cause behind a disease and focus instead on the physiological expression. Expression is often the effect and not the cause, and as long as the cause remains untreated, a pathological expression can remain (either in its original expression or as a manifestation of something else).

A perversion originating in either the anatomy, the mechanics, the physiology, and/or the pathology results in an alteration of all the others. It affects how one structure, hard or soft, interacts with another. While we always go back to the anatomy, we are interested in the interplay between structures, hard or soft. It is not enough to examine a joint in isolation and simply *know*. Of course, a firm knowledge regarding the structure and function of that joint is necessary, but the joint's true significance osteopathically is its relationship to other structures, proximally and/or distally. This is realized through our understanding of polygonal mechanics, which will be further discussed in the following chapters.

Physiology and pathophysiology are closely related. A *pathophysiology* is either a hypo- or a hyper-physiological expression. While we are always making new discoveries concerning the depth and breadth of these subjects, it is difficult to unequivocally say that this one element or another is being affected by osteopathic treatment. One can posit educated guesses about what is being affected and how, but the truth is that there always remains a grey area. Again, what can be observed, altered, and measured is the collective mechanics. If the hypo- or hyper-physiology has been positively modified by the reintegration of proper mechanics, physiological expression is returned to normal. To prepare the reader for how this can be done, the next chapter will begin discussion of the *what* of collective mechanics. From there we will venture into *why* (and ultimately *how*) it is used in osteopathic treatment. Before we consider these interrogatives, we will re-evaluate a global view of the quadrants that divide the axial skeleton.

2.3 The T-Lines

If we are to remain Stillian in our approach, we cannot (and should not) rush headlong into our assessment of osteopathy without discussing mechanics. The previous sections have mentioned the relationship between the anatomy and mechanics as ways of understanding normal and pathological processes in the body. It has been established that the mechanics are the objective element in our findings, both before and after treatment, whereby the reintegration and stabilization of structures within the body yield positive physiological results. The monumental shift from this mechanical perspective relies on the emphasis of structure in the structure/function relationship in the body. In other words, it is the functional anatomy that directs the understanding of physiological outcomes. For example, if patients have a primary problem with their ankle and their gait is consequently affected—which leads to congestion in the liver, which then leads to compromised metabolic function—we do not attempt to treat the metabolic function. We cannot put our hands on the physiology directly; instead, if the site of the primary lesion is the ankle, we treat the ankle. This then restores the impeded gait, which subsequently restores the body's natural rhythms and coordination—which ultimately has a positive impact on all metabolic functions, including those of the liver.

How do we determine, though, if it really is the ankle that is causing the problem? What if it was the shoulder? Or a group of ribs? What does collective mechanics look like? In other words, how do practitioners work through the body and determine a logical and correct osteopathic diagnosis? It is one thing to have an in-depth knowledge of anatomy, or a large battery of functional tests, or a detailed knowledge of physiology; it is another to put all of those tools together in a way that is inclusive, simple to use without compromising the complexity of the body, and effective in application. It is also a challenge to explain all of these elements in a way that practitioners can read and then apply in their practices. Therefore, this section of the book is broken down into different frameworks from which to read the body. One overlays the other and each can be used by practitioners to spiral in and out from a global understanding of a lesion pattern to one that is more local. We start by discussing the first layer with the T-lines. With Collective Mechanics, practitioners can use a method of differential diagnoses that hovers between modes of knowledge and assessment regarding normal and abnormal functions of the anatomy. The vitalistic expressions of the anatomy are crucial; they provide information on the body's ability to strive for health through all its compensatory mechanisms.

The use of T-lines provides practitioners with a quick visual and motion assessment that includes two horizontal lines, one from acromion to acromion for the Upper T-line, and from the top of one iliac crest to the other for the Lower. These two lines are bisected by a vertical line. This vertical line can be categorized into two essential divisions where the posterior line (the spine) has neurophysiological influence, and where the ventral line is fascial. Taken all together, practitioners can glean a global snapshot of sagittal and coronal lesion patterns. Most important, these lines provide a blueprint for treatment so that correction is always directed in reference to something else. In its simplest form, if there is a declination of the right shoulder, for instance, the goal is to elevate it so that this line is level again. If there is too great a fixed flexion where there should be extension along the vertical line, then that is what needs to be corrected so that each spinal curve can balance the other and function, collectively, as a true spinal organ.

These lines also let practitioners know if there exists a healthy compensation, a topic we will discuss in more detail in the Treatment section of the book. For now, it is enough to understand that there is essentially a declination in the upper and lower T-lines in the same direction. This could be an indication that more serious investigation is required when determining the seat of dysfunction in the pathology of afflicted patients. These lines also provide reference for what practitioners find in their palpation. If there is an uncompensated pattern, practitioners can predict what kinds of lesions they can expect when palpating and motion testing; the pattern will be reflected in all tissues of the body, whether fascial, muscular, ligamentous, boney, and/or organic. This will provide landmarks of information to practitioners, an essential part of administering treatment that considers the stabilization of corrective efforts.

With the inclusion of this simple tool, practitioners are better equipped to determine relationships between the upper and lower girdle, as well as the spine that runs vertical to them, in an orderly and efficient manner. On palpation, they are able to evaluate the tissue texture, the type of lesion, and how long it has persisted. Of course there is more to this process (as will be discussed), but for now practitioners can consider this expository framework to observe the pathogenesis of diminished somatic and organic physiological functions.

It Is about Correlation

Above all else, Collective Mechanics is a way of mapping the functional anatomy that is useful to the clinician. It is a model that follows Still's recommendations to look at the anatomy first and last, and it does so in a manner that is clinically relevant to the practitioner. It is easy to get lost in abstract theoretical models that cannot be measured through direct palpation and coordination of lines of force (be they hard or soft), or in an endless discussion of the physiology with little relevance to the application of treatment. While interesting to ponder, neither queries do well for providing a logical way of proceeding through the body with measurable outcomes. Operators must be able to quantify their findings through a series of differential diagnoses, which can then be applied throughout each course of treatment. To be sure, our discussion on mechanics is not to take the place of the anatomy or even the physiology; it is to support our ability to palpate, sequence a treatment that is efficient and effective, and to do so in a manner that liberates both practitioner and patient. It is through these methods that the body lets its own self-healing and self-regulating features take hold. The constitution and vitality of the individual improves as the practitioner assists in liberating the structures in lesion.

Knowing that the mechanics we discuss directly correlate to the anatomy of the human body, we can apply our principles to see how function is integrative and reflective of structure. Harkening back to our earlier discussion on palpation, this is to teach practitioners that the lesion resides in the passageways between structures. An understanding of how systems are interconnected and interdependent yields a better ability to identify abnormality between these connections. The more that junior practitioners employ this understanding, the better their functional comprehension of the body will be. Even if the names of structures are forgotten, the picture of the anatomy and how it is supposed to function will remain in the mind's eye—and it is this image that will benefit the patient.

Qualities of Healthy Mechanics

Let us begin by first discussing some qualities of healthy mechanics so that we, by way of deduction, have an understanding of unhealthy mechanics. First, all structures should have elasticity and plasticity within their physiological ranges of motion. Second, the body should work in a collective, integrated fashion. Third, the first and second conditions promote an environment for a healthy neurophysiology. In short, all health and adjustments to health are dependent on the qualities of proper mechanics in order to promote proper neurophysiological function. We will now introduce the next level of framework by focusing our attention on the coronal plane. From this vantage point we can establish a *functional* versus *dysfunctional* mechanical picture.

The Four Quadrants

As we note in Figure 1, practitioners should remember that bones in osteopathy are the framework on which we base our correlates, and that when we are discussing collective mechanics, we are really addressing the axial skeleton and all its relationships. As we examine the axial skeleton more locally, we require a model for assessment that allows the somatic and organic fields to be analyzed in a manageable way, one that adheres to our mechanical premise. To do this, we divide the axial skeleton into four quadrants on the coronal plane. The T-lines still exist in this model, forming the top and bottom horizontal lines. The centre horizontal line, which is bisected by the vertical line of the spine, is placed at what will be referred to as the primary pivot at D11/12 dorsally and the epigastric fossa ventrally. These are the sites for communication and integration of the central nervous system (CNS) on both the dorsal and

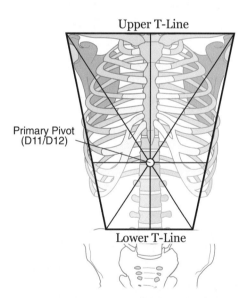

FIG. 1: Here we see the axial skeleton divided into four quadrants on the coronal plane. The T-lines form the top and bottom horizontal lines, and the centre horizontal line is at the level of the primary pivot (D11/12) dorsally, and the epigastric fossa ventrally.

ventral side of the body in relation to the spinal cord, the sympathetic chain, and the splanchnic nerves that form the epigastric, superior and inferior mesenteric, gastric, and renal plexuses. This site is also level with the adrenal glands, which have autonomic and endocrine influence for many normal physiological functions (such as the regulation of vasomotion). These functions (as will be discussed when the concept of polygonal mechanics is introduced) receive communications from many somatic structures, including the fascia of the psoas and the crux of the diaphragm.

From a diagnostic perspective, it is straightforward to visualize where each of the four boxes should be, with the upper and lower girdle (the upper and lower quadrants) integrated and coordinated with the primary pivot at its centre point. On the somatic side, natural and gravitational forces that impact the body are better received through its collective mechanics. On the organic side, each organ is able to function in its quadrant if the circulatory, nervous, and lymphatic systems are unrestricted by torsions or strains through the axial skeleton, and the overall physiological processes run smoothly. The body, in its eloquence, literally communicates that good symmetry equals, for the most part, good physiological function.

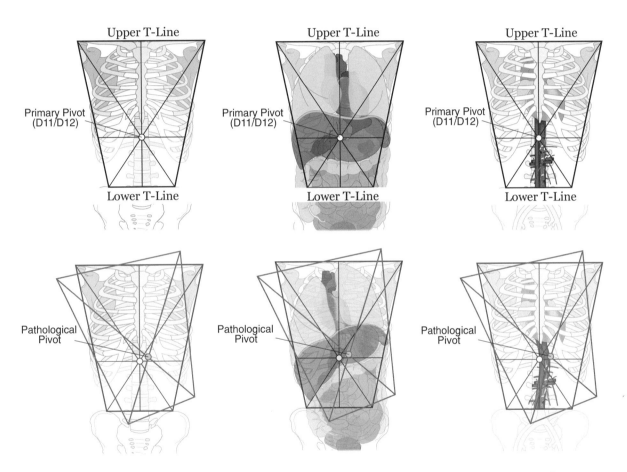

FIG. 2: Here we see the affect caused by asymmetry through the quadrants, and discoordination between the upper and lower girdles throughout the primary pivot. With the primary pivot off of its proper axis, a new mechanical pathological pivot is placed onto other structures, such as a rib head (*left*). In the visceral field, the pathological pivot point can create lesioning within the liver/gallbladder field or the stomach/spleen field. The abnormal forces encourage congestion throughout the organ field, for example, when the right lung compresses the liver (*centre*). The translation of force across the abdominal aorta not only affects the fluid dynamics of the system, but also the prevertebral plexuses of the autonomic nervous system. Tension from the pathological pivot point shown above (*right*) may create abnormal function of the celiac and superior mesenteric plexuses in particular, affecting digestion and elimination functions.

If, however, the quadrants are not symmetrical, and the upper and lower girdle are not integrated collectively through the primary pivot (as in Figure 2), all the systems that were in optimal working order now have to contend with abnormal forces permeating the somatic field on the one hand and the physiological field on the other. In such a case, the primary pivot is shifted off its proper axis, and the right lung descends over the liver. With the strain on the lung and compression on the liver, it stands to reason that there would be altered physiological function to both organs, which would then pathologize the regulatory and delivery systems to which they are connected.

This is a simple example on a two-dimensional plane, but if we consider Figure 3 and the typical spinal coupling in the dorsal and lumbar spine, there will be a torsional influence through unilateral or bilateral flexion extension. Now the tension and the compressive forces acting on these organs are further complicated by the additional strain assailing from the outside through the limbs.

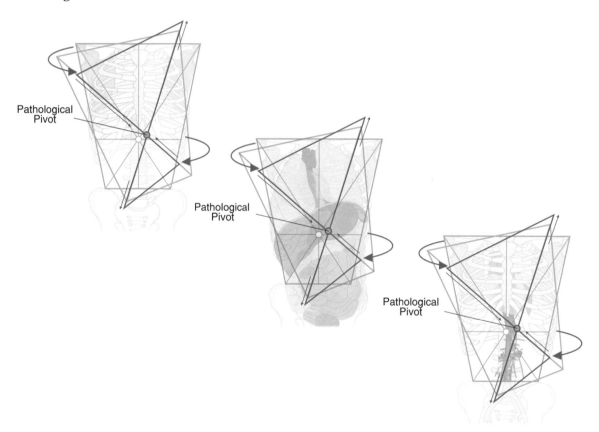

FIG. 3: Here a torsional influence brought about by a typical spinal coupling in the dorsal and lumbar spine has been added. The tension and compressive forces acting upon the organs is further complicated by the added strain coming from the outside, through the limbs.

Some Considerations of the Upper and Lower Limbs

Let's consider for a moment how the lower limb becomes part of the pathological lesion pattern, further compromising how the body deals with asymmetry in the four quadrants. Due to the asymmetrical shift at D11/12, one limb will express tension and the other compression. This mechanical lesion can also lead to a difference in vascular distribution between one leg and the other. With this in mind, it would be logical to assume there would also be a change in the physiological (not just fluid) makeup of these structures, which would then influence other parts of the body, whether somatic and/or organic. There are numerous mechanical influences that would allow practitioners to explore different compression zones (be it hard or soft tissue) that could alter fluid dynamics in addition to the aforementioned changes. That is why having a sequential, layer-by-layer approach is so important. Once the lesion pattern is identified, we must know what to do about it—and that strategy is derived from palpation.

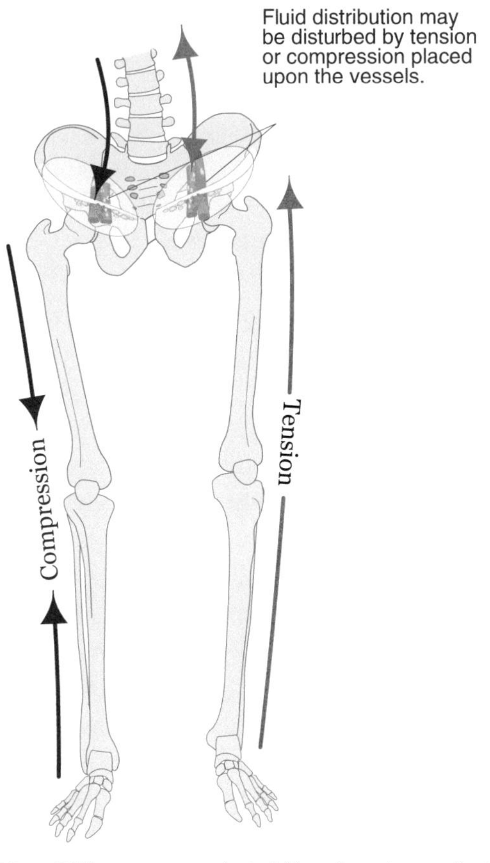

Fluid distribution may be disturbed by tension or compression placed upon the vessels.

Compression

Tension

FIG 4: With an asymmetrical shift at the primary pivot, a limb will express tension and the other compression. This mechanical lesion may lead to a difference in vascular distribution between one leg and the other.

Practitioners should be able to anticipate correlations between the lower and upper limbs in a similar away. In a common compensated pattern, practitioners often find one shoulder anterior and the other posterior, which can affect the neurovascular supply to and from the head, to the lung and heart field, and to the primary pivot at D11/12. For example, as the anterior shoulder drops off the thoracic wall, it compresses the axillary and subclavian vessels at the sternal end, causing a pivot of the clavicle that can then influence the carotid vessels to the head. The brachial plexus, the lower and middle cervical ganglia, and the stellate ganglia (bridging the cervical and thoracic sympathetic chain), are altered due to changes on the vascular demands invoked by the lesion. This has a strong influence on the vasomotor centres that cause irregularity in heart function, blood pressure, and respiration. The strain on the heart is made further evident by the mechanical swing of the girdle favouring one side over the other, creating an alternated physiological circulatory pattern. More specifically, this mechanical discord affects the potential physiological functioning of the heart owing to an asymmetry between the hard and soft tissues of the upper girdle and the structures beneath them.

With respect to endocrine function, the asymmetry of the shoulder girdle can cause strain across the anterior tissue of the neck, including the thyroid gland. Together with irregular vasomotion, the production and distribution of thyroid hormone can be altered, triggering any number of effects distal to the central point of origin, and even impacting remote regions of the entire body.

Compensation Patterns within This Model

In looking at the asymmetry between the upper and lower quadrants with a shift at the primary pivot and/or through outside influence via the upper and/or lower limbs, practitioners are able to recognize "patterns of compensation" identified by Gordon Zink, D.O., F.A.A.O.[1] As Zink explains, practitioners should detect more than the four basic patterns outlined in the standard compensation model, where we have common or uncommon compensated patterns, as well as uncompensated patterns to either the left or the right. By using the T-lines, practitioners have a global frame of reference for both assessment and correction; by using quadrants, they have a more local perspective while still being able to observe the compensation pattern with the primary pivot at D11/12. This primary pivot is joined by two other key pivots at the cervicothoracic (CT) and lumbosacral (LS) junctions.

Having a way to spiral in and out of the mechanics has profound clinical advantages, as we can consider each quadrant in digestible ways to establish a collective, differential diagnosis through these key junctions and quadrants. As a consequence, through the application of treatment these four quadrants and two torsional lines give us eight directions with axes and planes that provide a blueprint for observing how the body can move. If we then apply this understanding to what the body *can* do, we have the beginnings of a differential structural diagnosis by noting what the body *cannot* do. Treatment can then be targeted at those areas so that the body is restored to its dynamic balance, both functionally and physiologically. In terms of procedure, we can assess and motion test each of the four quadrants with our osteopathic structural diagnosis, and then, depending on the degree of lesion patterns found, use each of the limbs to help coordinate and integrate treatment for the body.

[1] Dr. Zink taught at the University of Osteopathic Medicine and Health Sciences at Des Moines, Iowa, and was an excellent clinician, who noted an alternating postural patterns that show opposing lines of influence between key transition areas in the body.

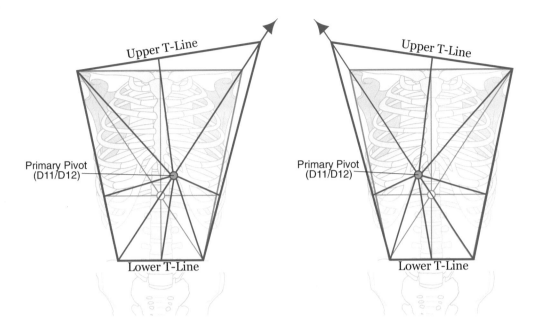

Forces directed through the long lever of the arm to affect the upper quadrants.

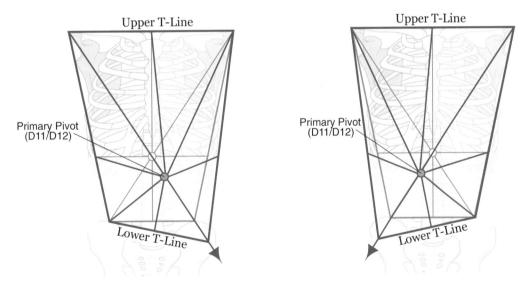

Forces directed through the long lever of the leg to affect the lower quadrants.

FIG. 5: Using functional anatomical connections between each of the four limbs and their corresponding quadrant will affect the alignment of the upper and lower girdles, as well as the primary pivot, through forces applied using the limb as a long lever.

The Sagittal Plane

When looking at the coronal plane (as illustrated on the prior page), it is easy to see each quadrant and imagine their movements on that plane. However, as we introduced in Figure 3, we know there are torsional movements from anterior to posterior on diagonal lines that complicate the matter. We must always remember that the body is three-dimensional—and so are its lesions. Now that we have seen how the body compensates on the coronal plane, we will consider how the anterior/posterior pitch and balance of the body compensates through flexion/extension.

In Figure 6, the reader will notice several pivots in the body that, when balanced in line with one another, allow the body to function optimally under natural and gravitational forces (both statically and dynamically). When these lines are in order, the head carriage is in an ideal position for the higher centres in the brain to best direct and distribute their orders for health. When the head is not sitting correctly on its pivot in the upper cervical complex, however, the body has difficulty determining where it is situated in its environment. This is because the proprioceptive systems are not functioning congruently with one another. Such incongruence amounts from these systems' perversion of collective mechanics as observed in relation to the lines of force acting on the body. As a consequence, the mechanico-physiological aspects of the lesion can only create physiological discord.

If we could directly adjust the higher centers to these newly altered mechanics, our work might be easier. Unfortunately, this type of direct adjustment is unlikely in this scenario; we instead affect these centers through the rest of the body, at which point the body is brought back to a neutral position so that the mechanical-pathological loop can be arrested. We achieve these corrections by way of two central pivots (the upper cervical complex and the coxofemoral joints) that should be lined up with one another from the sagittal view. One effective way to understand this position is to use the anatomy as our guide. In doing so, we determine the thoracolumbar junction, or primary pivot at D11/12, as the seat of stability that should be established to bring these structures into better alignment. If we survey the large moves below D11/12, we note that the primary motion is on the sagittal plane, providing flexion/extension. This includes the lumbar spine and the lower limbs. The upper limbs follow this flexion/extension rule, albeit the shoulder, like the hip, allows for circumduction, despite the fact that the thorax follows motion about the vertical axis from the primary pivot. The cervical spine is a soft tissue curve that functions as a combination of the lumbar and thoracic spine, allowing for sidebending/rotation to the same side in flexion/extension/neutral positions.

If the baseline is misaligned at the coxofemoral joints, so too will be the transition of forces through the lumbars and into the TL junction. The misalignment will affect not only the sagittal pitch of the body on its pivots, but also the position of the shoulder girdle as the body fights

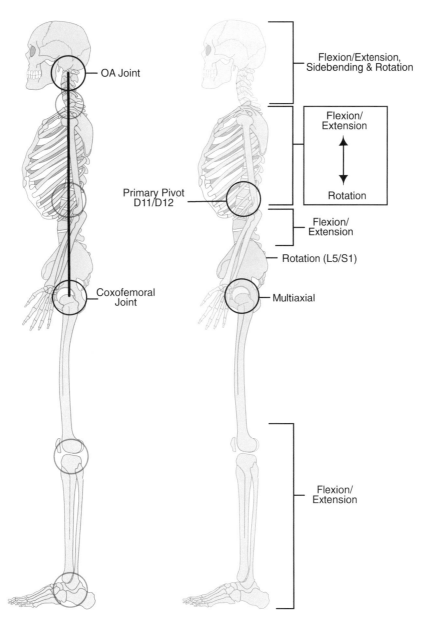

FIG. 6: Two central pivots that should be lined up with one another from the sagittal view—the upper cervical complex, and the coxofemoral joints.

Primary motion:
- Ankle/Knee - Flexion/Extension
- Coxofemoral - Multiaxial
- L5/S1 - Rotation
- Lumbar Spine - Flexion/Extension
- D11/D12 (Primary Pivot) - Rotation
- Lower Thoracic Spine - Rotation
- Upper Thoracic Spine - Flexion/Extension
- Cervical Spine - Flexion/Extension/Sidebending/Rotation

to keep balance for its higher centres to run correctly. For example, if the posture is posterior, the scapulothoracic joint will internally rotate to use the upper limbs as counterweights. If there is an anterior posture, the scapulothoracic joint will pull the thorax back, creating a separational strain on the vertebral column because of the flexion it induces—which then induces compression on the mediastinum and the sternum ventrally. This is what is known as a *kyphotic posture*. If there is a longstanding kyphotic posture, there will be a change in the fibrotic nature of the longitudinal ligaments. When the posterior longitudinal ligament thickens, it stops the spine from coming back into extension. The ribs will be "exhaled" in this position, up on the posterior surface, and down ventrally. The tension on the costosternal margins in this case is tremendous. The soft tissue changes in accordance to this position as the rhomboids will pull back; this causes external rotation of the shoulder (which involves the rotator cuff complex), and will then shorten the carrying angle of the upper limb. In either postures, we only need to focus on the vasomotor output and the diameter of the vessels in the upper limbs, the thorax, and all that it houses to search for the cause of any number of pathophysiological states.

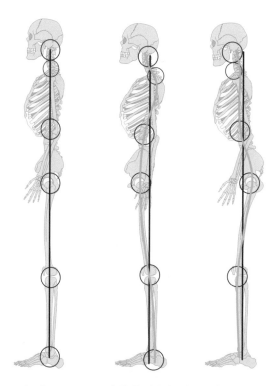

FIG. 7: A comparative illustration between neutral (*left*) and the changed transition of forces through the body in the sagittal plane caused by altered position of the baseline. With the coxofemoral joints translated anteriorly (*centre*), the scapulothoracic joint will pull the thorax back. With the coxofemoral joints translated posteriorly (*right*), the scapulothoracic joint internally rotates using the upper limbs as counterweights.

This illustration can be taken further if we remember that the seat of stability is not set, particularly if there is compression on the right lower limb due to sidebending to the right in the lumbar spine. As an example, the angulation and tension of the piriformis is modified as it passes from the anterior surface of the sacrum through the static notch to the greater trochanter, altering the force permeating the pelvis as a result of that lumbar sidebend. The change in angulation can cause fibrosity in the fascia over the left sacroiliac (SI) joint, which can potentially affect the sacral plexus. This is a key point in osteopathic thinking, for rather than looking only at the area of pain or pathology, we note that there is a sequela in the lesion.

Mechanically, the lumbar lesion is perpetuating the sacral discord. That discord is what affects the piriformis, which affects the position of the hip, for instance, and its external rotation. The sidebending from the lumbar spine then creates an uneven distribution between both legs and an external rotation of one of them. This has a potential effect on the autonomics of the left SI joint, which could then impact the descending colon. A disruption in the elimination cycle might then create a toxic environment in the body. With a distortion of either the kyphotic or extension positions of the thorax above, the pliability and functioning of the lungs could be compromised, further adding to the toxicity levels (which could be noted in the quality of the skin), and resulting in any number of possible respiratory conditions.

Taken further, this example then shows that a displaced pelvic girdle (owing to a lumbar sidebend) can produce a shear from one hip to the opposite shoulder, and potentially initiate a cascade effect on the lungs, heart, liver, and digestive functions. What is more important to take from this exercise, however, is that the limbs are really extensions of the visceral field and that osteopathic care provides treatment for innumerable conditions. By setting the upper and lower girdles, we are affecting the higher centres of the brain and allowing the full expression of health and wellbeing to reflect itself in the collective mechanics of the body.

Conclusion

Although we employ terms like Collective Mechanics, it is not our intention to rewrite osteopathy. Rather, our goal is to revive the Stillian perspective by shedding light on what might otherwise be considered an outdated concept—and we do this by returning to the anatomy. By employing terms such as "Collective Mechanics," what we are really talking about are mechanics themselves; the new name is simply a device to make the subject more intelligible for readers. With a firm understanding of a progressive (or layered) approach to mechanics, practitioners will be able to contemplate an array of connections not discussed here directly, but that are nevertheless part of the concepts we have introduced. These findings will reveal themselves through clinical experience with this model, and allow for osteopathic discussions whose centripetal point is to find better ways of addressing the lesion.

2.4 From Quadrants to Polygons

A Blessing and a Curse

The notion that our mechanics are based on functional anatomy is both a blessing and a curse for the purposes of presenting this material. It is a blessing in that we are providing a collective way of observing the body that is very effective in rendering intelligent diagnoses and treatment. It is a curse for the same reason, as we must find a way of explicating the anatomy in a layered, progressive approach that is at once comprehensible and true to its integrative nature. As we now move from the four quadrants to a discussion of polygons, it should be noted that we already started moving in this direction in the previous chapter. This kind of overlap is intentional: our method in outlining these approaches is to create a tapestry of understanding that will form a three-dimensional picture of the body.

One key point in our discussion is that when we talk about the mechanics, we are not only talking about the construction and mobility of the skeletal structure. We are trying to present a layered approach to the body that works from the boney tissue, to the soft tissue, and to everything in between (including the viscera). The body is a dynamic unit of function that is continually adapting to its internal and external environments. Histological alterations and changes in neurovascular systems in all tissues happen on a continual basis, not just at the boney level, but also at the ligamentous, the muscular, and the fascial. These alterations can be caused by mechanical and/or physiological influences. The problems many practitioners face when differentiating between the two are as follows: first, they do not acknowledge in their diagnosis the alterations in these matrixes of tissues, and therefore are unaware of the alteration in function (and the responsibilities of these tissues) as a result of these factors. Second, even if practitioners do find a key lesion and correctly identify its holding pattern, they do not have the patience and wisdom to work through the layers of tissue in a way that works with the body. As a consequence, they become fixated on a lesion without knowing the correct way to interact with it.

With the points above taken into consideration, we want to ensure that our approach to the mechanics is nuanced while also offering insight into the types of lesioning that can be expected (and why). Such an approach will provide clues for treating key lesion patterns. Sometimes they need to be treated distally and at other times proximally; sometimes they are treated with great intensity on the barrier and at other times not. With time, education, and experience, much of what is discussed in these pages, if integrated into practice, will encourage a more balanced approach where practitioners can rally confidence in their treatment plans.

From Quadrants to Polygons

To this point in our discussion, we have considered the four quadrants as an organizing and diagnostic tool, whereby we are able to transition from a global to a more local perspective. This capacity to transition from global to local offers a way of assessing lesion patterns related to the upper and lower T-lines, as well as a central vertical line down the vertical axis. Now we will make the quadrants more dynamic by overlaying a polygonal model (see the diagram below). There are many ways we can discuss polygon mechanics based on the quadrant mod-

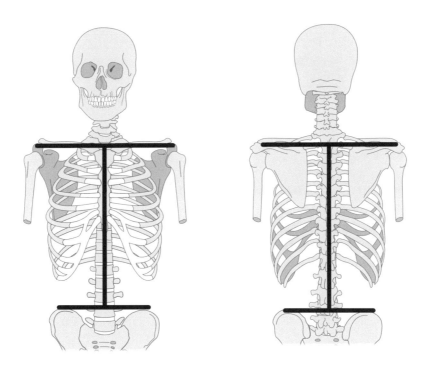

FIG 8: *Hard lines.* Consisting of the central motor line (spine) and the upper and lower T-lines.

el, and we have explored some of these ways in the last chapter. Now we add another layer to the foundation already set. To begin, though, we need to classify the types of lines with which we are working.

First, we have our hard (bony) lines. These consist of the motor line (or the spine), and the upper and lower T-lines. Each of these hard structures serves a specific function that is important for us to consider during assessment and treatment. The motor line contains, of course, the spine and its neurophysiological influence. The T-lines are horizontal lines that connect the limbs to the axial skeleton and function as pumps that aid in fluid and air dynamics. These lines influence—and are influenced by—soft tissue lines (which we will address in a moment). They are also responsible for the coordination and stabilization of ambulation and include major muscle groups that span from the limbs to the axial skeleton. With this understanding, we have a blueprint of what we are adjusting, and if the body does not conform to this ideal position, further investigation is warranted. This centripetal exploration comes from being able to move in and out of the quadrants while also considering the influence to and from the limbs down to the primary pivot of D11/12.

If we look again at the quadrants, we can extend a line off each corner to represent a limb. The symmetry between one limb and another, as well as the limbs' range and quality of motion, reflects lesioning to and/or from the axial frame. In either case, of greatest significance are the major muscles that come from the limbs and T-lines to intersect at D11/12. Of course, there are many aspects of myology we could include in our discussion, but for the sake of the scope of this work, we will limit the groupings to the major muscles so as to build a clear picture in the reader's mind. Larger anatomical features have a larger responsibility in the body; therefore, it makes sense to assess and correct substantial components prior to dealing with the minutiae (or structures).

Along the ventral surface of the body, from caudad to cephalad, we find psoas and the pectoralis muscles. From the dorsal surface of the body, from cephalad to caudad, we find trapezius and quadratus lumborum. There are other reflexive muscle groups that include the rotators and stabilizers of the upper and lower limbs, and the importance of these muscle groups is dictated by the functional anatomy. They are large, strong muscles that tether the external frame of the arms and girdles to the axial, internal frame of the motor line. Should there be lesioning in and along these muscles, the T-lines (the horizontal hard lines) will be augmented, which will then distort the position and mobility of the spine (the central line).

Even when these lines distort and the symmetry between the quadrants is lost because of either internal or external factors, the body will attempt to balance itself through compensa-

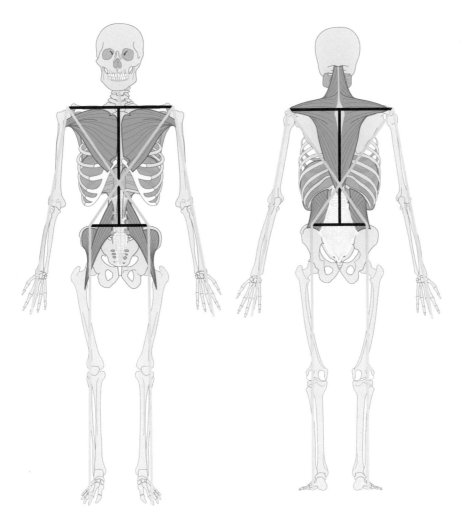

FIG. 9: Here the major muscles that come from the limbs and T-lines and intersect at D11/12 are added on top of the hard lines. Muscles of interest include psoas and pectoralis major on the ventral side, and trapezius and quadratus lumborum on the dorsal side.

tion—but its efforts are altered both statically and dynamically by the lesion. A lesion in one part of the body affects the whole; in this particular case, the lesion emanates through these lines that work along torsional strains (from the upper polygon to the lower polygon), and converge at the mechanical and physical centre of motion for the body. But how, exactly, does this process unfold?

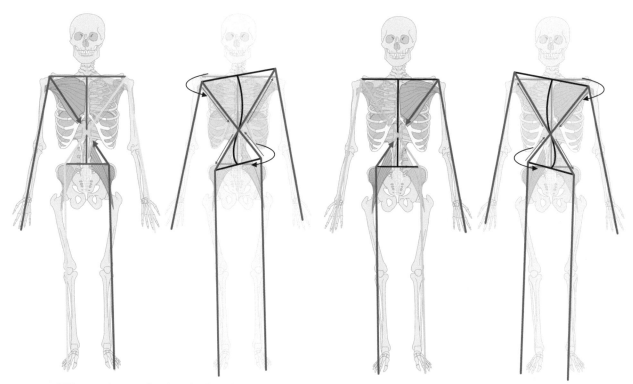

FIG. 10: Here, torsional strains from the upper polygon to the lower polygon are shown on the ventral lines between the psoas muscles and the contralateral pectoralis major.

Key Junctions

There are key junctions that aid in assessment and treatment when dealing with these two horizontal lines and the one vertical line. We already mentioned the primary pivot at D11/12 (TL), but practitioners must also consider the cervicothoracic junction (CT), the lumbosacral junction (LS), the bilateral pivots at the coxofemoral (CF) joints, and the upper cervical complex (OA/AA). First, we will discuss the importance of the latter two and then correlate them with the former.

When the OA/AA, the TL, and the CF joints are in line mechanically, the body does a much better job, neurologically, with its regulatory processes along the higher centres and the medulla. In this instance, the nervous system is aided in its regulatory functions from D11/12 (a centre of physiological motion). Here, the ventral ganglia travels from the posterior spine to the ventral fossa, where it spreads to coordinate visceral reflexes in the organ field. With respect to the vascular system, D11/12 is also the centre for the adrenal glands, whose axes and neurology interface with the cardiopulmonary system neurologically. Mechanically, D11/12, or the primary pivot, as we call it, also harnesses the primary motion of the upper polygon, which is sidebending/rotation and flexion/extension in the lower polygon.

Bilateral Hinging

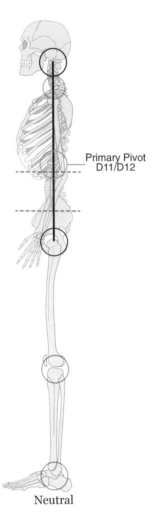

Primary Pivot
D11/D12

Neutral

FIG. 11: Here we can see the body in a relative neutral alignment, with a vertical line from the upper cervical complex to the coxofemoral joints. Two horizontal divisions isolate the lumbar spine. Within this division are the primary joints for flexion/extension. Sidebending/rotation comes to a point at the primary pivot.

Although it is true that D11/12 mediates the primary motions of the upper polygon (sidebending/rotation) with the lower polygon (flexion/extension), it can be difficult for practitioners to know what to do with this information. To help, we will explain how the anterior and posterior curves achieve balance. If we look at Figure 11, we will note a vertical line from the upper cervical complex to the coxofemoral joints from the lateral view. When the pitch of the CF joints or the OA/AA complex are correct, the body remains relatively neutral. If, however, we find alterations in the lower T-line (CF joints), the body will have to compensate to bring the upper cervical complex back in line (and vice versa). The body attempts this by altering the positioning of the anterior curves, which can result in strains on the dorsal spine.

Also depicted in Figure 11, we have made two horizontal divisions isolating the lumbar spine to show that the sidebending/rotation comes to a point at the primary pivot. The lower dividing line displays where the primary joints for flexion/extension exist in the lower limb. Should there be a change in the pitch of how the head of the femur fits in

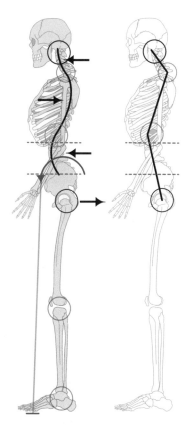
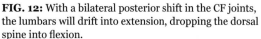
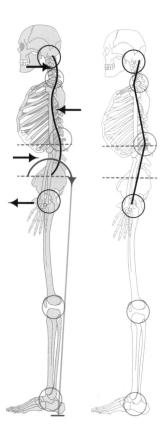

FIG. 12: With a bilateral posterior shift in the CF joints, the lumbars will drift into extension, dropping the dorsal spine into flexion.

FIG. 13: Here the CF joints are positioned anterior bilaterally, which adjusts the lumbar spine into a flexed position, putting the dorsal spine into extension.

the acetabulum, the lumbar spine will have to compensate to address the shift in the position of the baseline to support the proper position of the upper cervical complex. For example, as we see on the left in Figure 12, if there is a bilateral posterior shift in the CF joints, the lumbars will drift into extension, dropping the dorsal spine into flexion. In Figure 13 on the right, the CF joints are positioned anterior bilaterally, which adjusts the lumbar spine into a flexed position, putting the dorsal spine into extension. This means that the function and position of D11/12 and the thorax are often affected by what is occurring in the anterior curves. The primary pivot cannot perform its function as the transition point between primary motions of sidebending/rotation and flexion/extension if the base is unstable. The seat of stability for mechanical and physiological activity in this area must be set by the correct positioning of the tissues that rely on its function. The attachment of the two psoas muscles positioned ventrally along the lumbar spine to the lesser trochanter make for ideal tension lines to tether the CF hinge for flexion/extension below and above to the D11/12 junction. If there is only one hip in lesion, however, the psoas will adjust for a unilateral glide at the CF joint in an attempt to stabilize the base; yet it can also do so effectively within the physiological range of compensation of the body.

Unilateral Hinging

After perusing the example of a bilateral compensation mediated by the lumbar spine, it should be obvious that a unilateral glide would cause a shortening of one psoas and a lengthening of another, allowing the lumbar spine to fall into unilateral flexion/extension. It should also be obvious how that unilateral torsion would then have the same but opposing effect on the dorsal spine at D11/12, which hinges in the opposite direction, forming a compensatory torsion. As long as the compensation is within normal physiological limits, health is maintained. Should the strain, however, become too great or too fixed, the compensation between the upper and lower polygon will become too pronounced, which can be noted in an asymmetry in the trapezius on the dorsal side.

If practitioners think analytically, they will see that the effects of the unilateral hinge on the soft tissue forms a continuous strain through large muscles that work oblique axes. The psoas extends from the trochanter to D11/12 in the lower polygon, and the trapezius continues from the primary pivot to the upper T-line. From the acromia, the inverted triangle pattern of the trapezius reverses as it continues to the occiput. Ventrally, the sternocleidomastoid mirrors the psoas, extending from posterior to anterior, to continue to help compensate for the unilateral hinge at the seat of stability. What we find here is a suspensory system of long myological lines that have mirrored relationships between transition zones. Noting changes to these structures can aid practitioners' entry into treatment by first addressing these long torsional patterns, and, in doing so, they can differentiate between the types of lesion perpetuating the pathological patterns (be it hard or soft tissue).

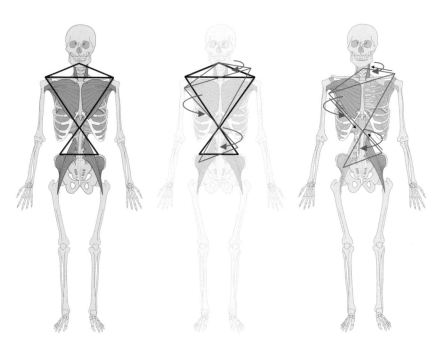

FIG. 14: The unilateral hinge on the soft tissue forms a continuous strain through large muscles that work oblique axes, including the psoas in the lower polygon, the trapezius in the upper polygon, and the trapezius from the upper T-line spanning towards the occiput (*centre*). The sternocleidomastoid mirrors the psoas, going from posterior to anterior, to continue to compensate for the unilateral hinge at the seat of stability (*right*).

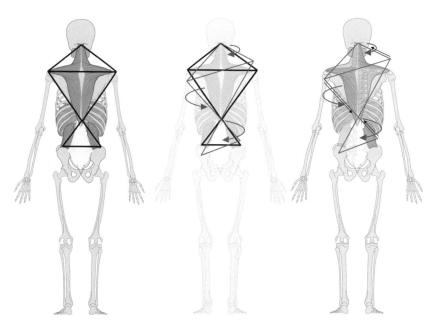

FIG. 14b: The unilateral hinge, dorsal view.

Differential Diagnosis between Hard and Soft Tissues

This is merely an introduction to polygon mechanics; how this model works with the functional anatomy can be further elucidated. Provided here is a clinical model premised on establishing testable results to better gauge the effectiveness of treatment. To do this, we will now analyze an example of how to use our current understanding of polygon mechanics in a differential diagnosis.

While continuing our focus on long oblique myological lines that operate within the soft tissue mentioned above, we can include both the pectoral muscles ventrally and the quadratus lumborum (QL) muscles dorsally. Borrowing from our Figure 14 illustrations, if the anterior pectoralis line is short on the right, there will be torsion toward the opposing direction on the opposite side. That torsion will travel through the thorax down to D11/12. The QL on the opposite will typically compensate with a contracture to help balance the polygons. In motion testing, we see this short pec inducing a sidebending/rotational coupling down to D11/12. If we then treat the soft tissue lateral line—that is, if the lesion remains at the central pivot and the tension on the QL did not change—we know that it is not a soft tissue lesion on the ventral side. The next logical step in our process is to determine if it is a hard or organic tissue lesion.

If, after removing the short pec line, the rotation at D11/12 is still present, we can test the motor line's deep intrinsic musculature and ligamentous structures. If the lesion persists after treatment has been applied in the areas of interest, we can test the kidney and the lower splanchnic nerves ventrally. We must also consider the position of distal structures, such as the innominates, which form the boney base of the lower polygon. With respect to mirrored structures in the upper polygon, we must remember that the cervical column mirrors the lumbar spine, and that the same approach, searching for neurophysiological correlates, is useful in establishing a diagnosis.

Once this area has been corrected, we can spiral out of the lesion the same way we went in, assessing the intrinsic boney lesion (proximal and distal) in relation to the reflex and the long myology. In working this way, we are able to rebalance these structures relative to the primary correction established by our differential diagnosis. According to this example, we began with the pec line under the assumption that it was in greater lesion with respect to the QL. (Bear in mind that we could have constructed this example from the QL to the pec.) From this understanding, beginning in either the upper or lower polygon, we are also able to use a differential approach with our understanding of collective mechanics to customize a method that spirals in and out of the lesion pattern in real time. Never are practitioners left wondering where to go next in their treatments; they simply read and react to the tissues and let the body be their guide.

Conclusion

One of the goals of this book is to present an approach that is neither "one size fits all" nor rooted in theory without clinical results. With that in mind, we have done our best to identify the major lines of force, hoping that readers will begin to think of their functional anatomy and fill in the blanks not covered in this introduction to the principles of mechanics and treatment. We hope that practitioners are thinking as much as they are reading, are beginning to ask better questions in their own approaches to diagnosis and treatment, and are starting to make decisions based on their deductive reasoning as much as their palpation. We will now further explain our argument for a collective approach to the body. In this next chapter, we continue our discussion of polygons and key lesions.

2.5 Polygons to Internal/External Frames and Key Lesions

A Point of Reference

As a pedagogical tool, this book relies on repetition and paraphrase to minimize confusion when delivering new material. To this end, we hope the more advanced reader sees the wisdom of our approach, for each time a point is reiterated in either the same or a different way, it is done to expand the breadth and depth of the osteopathic principles for all levels of practitioners. In this chapter we continue our discussion of the four quadrants and polygon mechanics. To deepen the reader's understanding of the material already covered, we use additional vocabulary that will help explain how we can identify key and supporting lesion patterns in the body. We will discuss the concepts of *internal* and *external frames* as a way of analyzing polygonal mechanics, and we will introduce other key junctions in the body apart from D11/12. In this chapter, these key transition zones will be regarded as rotatory hubs surrounded by a universal belt system. The universal belt system in this model is the spinal organ. This dynamic suspension system will then be juxtaposed by the effects of key lesions and their contributory lesions. This will, hopefully, alter the conventional barrier model and function of palpation during treatment, as well as change the way we perceive the spine and approach spinal treatment.

Where Have We Come From? Where Are We Going?

The image below should be referenced by readers in the context of what has been presented thus far. Readers should recognize the four quadrants and the two polygons (upper and lower). They will also see that we have three key pivots at the cervicothoracic (CT) junction, the thoracolumbar (TL) junction, and the lumbosacral (LS) junction. All of these elements will be essential to understanding the concept of key and secondary lesion patterns.

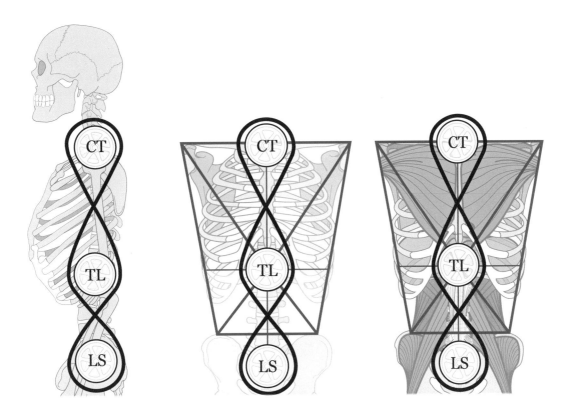

FIG. 15: The four quadrants and the two polygons (upper and lower) are shown in relation to the three key pivots at the cervicothoraco (CT) junction, the thoracolumbar (TL) junction, and the lumbosacral (LS) junction.

Review of the Barrier Model

We should recall briefly what was discussed with reference to the barrier model. The barrier is not a thing that we do something *to*; instead, it is something we interact *with* in order to restore proper communication between pathways in the regulatory systems of the body. As a consequence, we are interested in how the space between us and the lesion behaves. Distinguishing the type of lesion is the next step to determine the best mode of correction. As stated earlier, we have three main types of lesions under discussion: singular, chain, and complex. With any of these types there is a degree of fixation in the body that leads to compromised mechanical and physiological output. Our ability to palpate and understand the nature of the fixation and its secondary lines of influence are what determine our degree of success when identifying the cause of the dysfunction. If simply left to palpatory skills without an understanding of the collective mechanics of the body, practitioners can become confused about what is a key lesion and what is not. As practitioners' ability to palpate increases and a myriad of lesions leap into their hands, confusion can become frustration because knowing where to start and when to stop will be difficult.

Levels of Lesioning, Superficial to Deep

Consequently, it is common for junior practitioners to over-treat, over-stimulate, and overload the body, and thus inhibit its natural ability to find health. If, however, they are able to navigate the body and find different points that direct them to the primary lesion(s) and not lose themselves in the minutiae of what they are palpating, then a successful outcome (and practice) is more likely.

Why We Use Polygons and Where We Go from Here

The polygonal model, as it has been laid out thus far, is quite useful as both a diagnostic and corrective tool because it describes the anatomy along lines of force between hard and soft tissues. It gives us the opportunity to have something to adjust the body to, as Still suggests. Here, we see how the internal (motor) line and the external (lateral) lines interact and, ultimately, inform the treatment outcomes. This perspective is useful for delivering treatment that is effective and efficient, as it is based on the principle that the body is self-regulating and self-healing. Although this statement may seem obvious, it is often misunderstood due to differing concepts of correction. Oftentimes these concepts resemble orthopaedic practice rather than osteopathy.

This overlap of disciplines deserves elaboration because, as mentioned before, there are schools of osteopathy that fall into the category of orthopaedics, largely owing to their divergence from original Stillian principles. Hopefully it is apparent by now that we have done our best to return to a Stillian way of thinking about osteopathy. To this end, we do not treat the ankle in isolation and then the pelvis, just as we do not have a specialized treatment for asthma or measles. Nor do we impose a general treatment on the body for every session, as we instead work to give the body the best opportunity for health by using the mechanics as our schema. Our reason for doing this is to model the efficacy the patient expects by focusing the treatment on two principles: one mechanical and the other neurophysiological. Both take root in the osteopathic understanding of anatomy, which is applied with an integrative approach according to the laws that govern movement and health in the body. The applied anatomy that affects the neurophysiology is greatly influenced by the mechanical lines of force that determine the body's ability to function as intended. That is where and why the concepts and principles of the four quadrants and polygons were introduced; it is also why we must now extend our understanding of these ideas and repurpose them for the application of treatment.

Polygons as Internal and External Frames

Perspective is everything. The perspective we are cultivating here is through a clear but layered vocabulary that provides depth and nuance to our osteopathic understanding. How we view the body determines the quality of assessment, treatment, and the patient's reaction to treatment. For this section, therefore, we will refer to the lines in polygon mechanics as internal and external frame. It is recommended that readers keep the polygons in their mind's eye while studying this section and considering these images, for they are to be superimposed on one another. We use these terms to aid visualization of how both frames must remain parallel and synchronized to work effectively (similar to that of a door frame and a door). If they are not correctly adjusted to one another, the structure will not function as it should. The same is true of the entire body, as structure determines function.

The lateral lines from the upper and lower T-lines form the external frame, and the motor line/spinal organ consists of the internal frame. The body has the best chances at maintaining physiological balance when the mechanics are in order. Let us now revisit the polygons from this new perspective to see how the mechanics work, as it will broaden our later discussions.

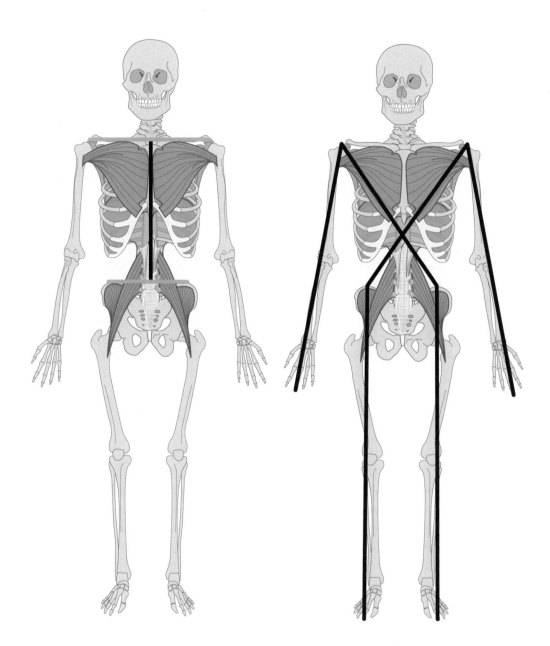

FIG. 16: The lateral lines from the upper and lower T-lines form the External Frame, and the motor line/spinal organ consists of the Internal Frame (*left*). The External Frame follows the limbs into the axial frame to D11/12 (*right*).

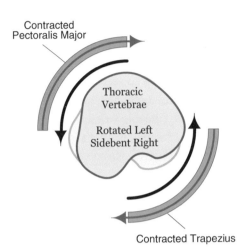

Contracted
Pectoralis Major

Thoracic
Vertebrae

Rotated Left
Sidebent Right

Contracted Trapezius

FIG. 17: The operator may globally address the External Frame in order to better determine the degrees of lesioning in the Internal Frame.

The operator should note that the External Frame may be compensating for the lesion pattern of the Internal Frame. In this case, the operator applies the principle of treating superficial to deep, addressing the soft tissue lines of the External Frame in order to see the deeper lesioning of the osseous Internal Frame.

The illustrated example above shows a left rotation throughout the thoracic vertebrae (osseous to Internal Frame). The soft tissue in the thorax from the External Frame compensates with a right torsion.

The external frame follows the limbs into the axial frame to D11/12, which means lesioning to and/or from this outer frame has influence to and from the spine. The internal frame can influence the external frame, but the primary lesioning along the spine has more to do with the health of the spinal organ and its autonomic and organic fields of influence. These frames are based on the functional anatomy. If practitioners work with this in mind, they have a way of reasoning through the body to find the cause of lesioning, as well as a method for systematically treating the body with the concepts of integration, coordination, and balance. This method applies to all the types of tissues that affect each of these frames. As a result, operators have a way of making sense of their palpation and can proceed with a Stillian perspective in mind.

If the two frames are regarded collectively, it is easy to see how they can be used in treatment. Once the tension is relieved off of the spine (the internal frame) by globally addressing the external frame, the operator can then better determine the degree of the lesion in the spine (whether it is a singularity, a chain, or a complex chain dysfunction). Our analysis, then, can progress in a global, local, and focal sequence. After globally liberating the superficial tissues that are connected to the external frame, we are able to work more locally on a region within a quadrant, and/or more focally on a segment in the spine. As we work more focally, we remain continually mindful of its impact on the external frame, and so our treatment protocol integrates the changes we make. This helps the body take on the intention of the treatment, raising the odds of success.

Adjusting to Relative Normal

The model we are using here indicates the normal (ideal) lines of the body. Our lines of force should be balanced, our internal and external frames aligned correctly, and our quadrants be in their respective places. In short, this arrangement provides the lines to which we adjust the body. The better we understand these concepts, the better our ability to recognize and adjust the abnormal to the normal. It also gives us license to see how the body has been influenced by Wolf's Law, making our universal model of the mechanics applicable to each individual's tendencies. This allows them to then regain their own potential for achieving an ideal state of structure and function. Therefore, our treatment approach is adjustive to a relative normal.

Major Pivots and Pulleys

With the concepts surrounding internal and external frames in mind, we can now show how they interact in a dynamic way that is based on the potentiality of lesioning within any individual. If we look at Figure 18, we see the upper and lower polygon as the external frame. To

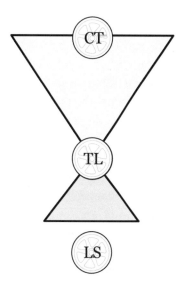

FIG. 18: The CT, TL and LS junctions are pulleys that are unified by the Internal Frame.

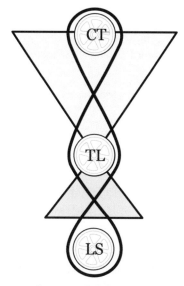

FIG. 19: *Belt Loop.* A belt loop around the pulleys shows the dynamic relationship between the Internal and External Frames. When the body is balanced, the tension on the belt is uniform and there is symmetry in position and motion of the upper and lower T-lines and the vertical line.

represent the CT, TL, and LS junctions (each a major transition zone) mechanically, we have superimposed cylinders or pulleys that are unified by the internal frame. Instead of depicting the motor line of the internal frame as a straight line, however, we have drawn a belt that loops around each of these pulleys to show the dynamic relationship between the internal and external frames. When the body is balanced, the tension on the belt is uniform and there is symmetry in position and motion of the upper and lower T-lines and the vertical line. This is the ideal that we seek when adjusting the patient, for these are natural places for the body to absorb and (re)distribute force to help maintain proper balance and neurophysiological function.

When these lines are not balanced, we see something interesting in how well this belt system works in relation to the T-lines. If there is a key lesion in the rib field, for example, as in Figure 20, we have a point of fixation. That point forms its own pathological pivot that augments the tension and position of the central belt, which means that, over time, it becomes an extra cylinder. The same belt, without changing its length, must loop around this new point. But in doing so, it pulls the T-lines of the polygons off their axes. The two frames, internal and external, are now no longer coordinated, as in Figure 21. With this altered position, we can see how the ambulation of the limbs are also affected. Now the quadrants are no longer balanced and a host of mechanical adaptations need to take place to abate any physiological degradation. For example, the strain from this new position places stress on baroreceptors and

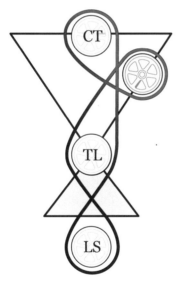

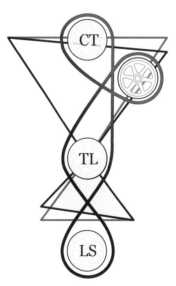

FIG. 20: *Key Lesion.* A key lesion is added to the rib field causing a fixation point. The fixation point becomes a pathological pivot that augments the tension and position of the central belt.

FIG. 21: *Effect on T-Lines & Polygons.* The belt remains the same length; thus the new fixation point causes the belt to pull the T-lines and polygons off their axes. This causes the internal and external frame to become uncoordinated.

chemoreceptors that then strain neurovascular output to maintain gas and fluid dynamics. If left untreated, the augmented mechanics stresses and weakens both the constitution and vitality of the body.

The Radiating Force of a Key Lesion

In Figure 22 we see that the primary fixation, or key lesion, creates a holding pattern of secondary lesions that facilitate its position. Because the body is a collective unit of function, a lesion is not necessarily localized to one area. Indeed, as new pivots, they form new lines of force that need to be abated, necessitating supportive points of fixation to keep the body dynamically balanced. Over time, they spread through the body, creating their own key pivots that allow the body to best stabilize itself through ambulation with its primary lesions. As a consequence, these secondary and tertiary lesions form a facilitating pattern. As primary fixations and the facilitating patterns reinforce one another, they form their own pathological belt system that is now in competition with the physiological belt system—the spinal organ. Now, we have two belts: one physiological and one pathological. Over time, one will take over the other and either lead to health or disease. We can see how proper mechanics and health can be compromised, as the influence of the fixation radiates and establishes itself over time. Add to this other competing lesions that form from other points of fixation with their own facilitating patterns and it is easy to see how difficult treatment can be, and why we often talk about teasing out the disease process through a course of osteopathic care.

The Radiating Force(s) of Correction

This idea of teasing out a lesion may sound well and good in theory, but it is how we put this theory into practice that gives it merit. It is clear, from what is mentioned above, that the goal of treatment should be to remove the primary point(s) of fixation and return coordination between the internal and external frames. We do this by motion testing the upper and lower polygon and palpating the most restrictive point of fixation. Then, as Figure 23 shows, we can see lines of force radiating to and from the lesion. At this point, everything we have highlighted about mechanics should be taken into consideration: we are attempting to return functional symmetry to each of the four quadrants; we are coordinating the upper and lower T-lines in relation to the internal frame; we are working, then, on all planes and axes of hard and soft tissue; and we are doing so by removing all facilitating patterns that might be connected to that lesion (due to the different corrective lines of force being applied by the

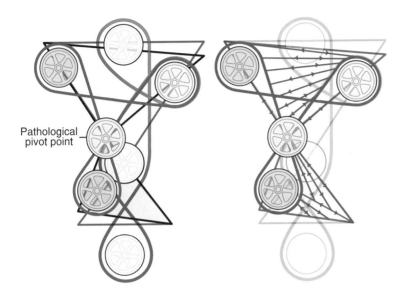

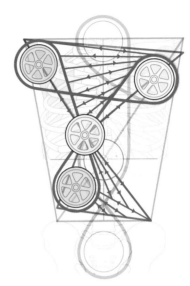

FIG. 22: *Holding Pattern.* The key lesion creates a holding pattern of-secondary lesions that facilitate its position. Primary fixations and the facilitating patterns reinforce one another, and the pathological belt system created competes with the physiological belt system.

FIG. 23: *Lines of Force.* Lines of force radiate to and from the lesion. We must attempt to return functional symmetry to each of the four quadrants.

operator). This is why osteopathy, in the classical sense, is not and cannot be orthopaedic, eclectic, or based on the whole body lesion theory. There is no one treatment for *condition A* or *condition B*; each are particular to an individuated complex of primary and facilitating lesion patterns that can only be addressed with an osteopathic understanding of mechanics, anatomy, and their principles.

Conclusion

With this knowledge, our discussion on the different types of lesions—singular, chain, and complex—make good sense as they are different degrees of primary points of fixation and facilitating patterns that keep the operator from getting lost in the minutiae of a pathology. All pathologies are dealt with by giving the body its best potential for curing itself by clearing any and all lesions that are obstructing it from doing its natural, innate job of finding health and longevity. At this point in the discussion on mechanics, we recommend students go back and re-read our discussion on the barrier model and the fully lesioned spine to help understand how the mechanics and manifestation of lesions inform one another. We will be later adding to this concept of key lesions by discussing primary, secondary, and tertiary lesions, as well as improving our abilities to differentiate between the qualities of tissue and how they correspond to different levels of lesioning (from superficial to deep). For now, we will take our current knowledge and apply it to a more focal understanding of spinal mechanics to address misconceptions on how the spine works as a collective unit of function. We will articulate the importance of the principle of global, local, and focal as it pertains to successful diagnosis and how it relates to the principle of correlation.

2.6 The Spinal Organ and the Buckled Arch

Where Do We Find the Ideal Anatomy?

When Still talks about having a living image of the anatomy in the mind's eye, he is referring to the ideal structure of the body as it should be, with symmetry and functionality throughout. But where do we locate this ideal? In an anatomy textbook? Perhaps, but discrepancies exist in varying anatomical ideation. We cannot base our methods on one text alone. This does not mean that we never consider anatomy books outside the discipline of osteopathy; such a declaration would run counter to the integrative approach we advocate. Yet it does mean that we follow the functional anatomy as represented in the collective mechanics. Indeed, the mechanics are the blueprint from which practitioners can derive meaning and adjust the body to its ideal. Again, remember that this model is particular to the individual. Everyone has these mechanical lines of reference and similar lines of force (either extending through the key pivots or being augmented by primary and secondary points of fixation), and for each individual, our adjustment is based on what we palpate in them.

We are now able to note the torsional forces that can affect the anatomy and the physiology dependent on it. Yet there is more to consider than just torsional twists between these two parts of the frame: we also have the spinal organ itself to assess and coordinate in relation to the collective mechanics. The forces that contribute to the osteopathic lesion include all planes. When we are talking about sidebending/rotation, we are discussing unilateral flexion/extension. Additionally, it is worth addressing how unilateral and bilateral lesions can result from a malpositioning of the spine. To comprehend this type of lesioning, the practitioner must see the spine for what it is: a collection of arches that ultimately act as a unified spring. That unified spring and its arches are influenced by its structure and function relationship. That structure/function relationship is to be considered within the principle of correlation with respect to the internal and external frames covered in the previous section. The entire relationship is also influenced by injury and augmented physiological function. We will focus, for a moment, on the internal frame with respect to its collective influence on the health of the patient.

Buckled vs. Compressed Arch

As we discuss matters of the spine, it is important that we proceed cautiously with our vocabulary. For instance, we would not want to characterize the spine as a stack of blocks—one segment on top of the other—as this is not an apt analogy. That is why we do not use the term "compression lesion" when addressing the spine, as it is not a vertical column but a series of arches. So when we talk about "arch mechanics" and "spinal lesions," we should be focusing on points where it can buckle into either flexion or extension. As we will discuss, this will most likely happen at either the top, the middle, or the bottom of the arch, all of which tend to receive the greatest load, and are typically regarded as transition zones from the primary motion mechanism of one curve to another.

As we discuss these transition zones, we will generally include the primary ones we have already covered as key pivots. With more time and exploration, readers may find others, but for our purposes it is enough to name the CT, TL, and LS junctions and the mid-position of each of these junctions. Most lesioning will present itself at these key junctions because motion characteristics change from an anterior/posterior on the vertical axis in these areas. The arch of each of these curves—the cervical, the dorsal, the lumbar, and the sacral—also juxtapose one another, from anterior to posterior. Let us now look more locally at each arch.

Three Points within the Arch: The Bow String Effect

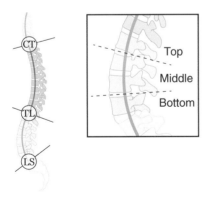

FIG. 24: Each curve, or arch, can be divided into three major sections: the top, middle, and bottom.

Each curve, or arch, can be divided into three—the top, middle, and bottom. The overlap between each arch matches the key transitions zones in our belt theory. Approached from a sagittal view, however, the three points of the arches can been seen with respect to their anterior/posterior relationship to one another. For the anterior curves, there will be two posterior divisions at either end functioning as key pivots, and one anterior portion bisecting them to form a minor pivot. For the posterior curves there is the inverse, particularly where there are two anterior divisions at either end, and one posterior portion bisecting. Each arch then has portions that triangulate with one another, where the mid-portion will naturally either drift anterior or posterior respective to its curve. In a healthy spine, the centre of gravity line will travel through each of the key transition zones.

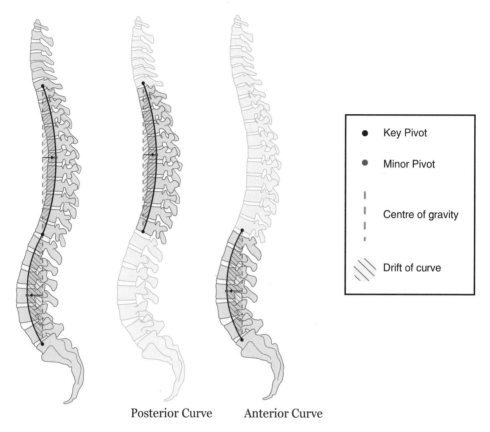

Posterior Curve   Anterior Curve

FIG. 25: *Anterior and posterior curves.*

As we must regard the spine collectively, we need to perceive its relations: first, we need to see how the triangulation points within each arch affects its position; and second, we need to see how changes in triangulation within each arch affects how the arches interact with one another. For instance, a flexion lesion in and around D6 might be driven by an extension lesion at D1 and D12. The way to deal with this lesion at D6 is to realize that, potentially, the arch has buckled owing to the extension pattern being driven by extension lesions in the anterior curves that are D1 and D12. In this way, the flexion lesion at D6 is addressed in relation to the whole spine where each curve is divided into three points of triangulation. These observations suggest that a treatment method be implemented to soften the anterior curves in order to change the position and functionality of D1 and D12, which then allows D6 to drift back to a more physiologically appropriate position.

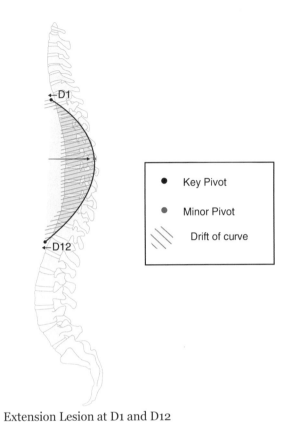

Extension Lesion at D1 and D12

FIG. 26: *Flexion lesion at D6 driven by extension lesions at D1 and D12.*

Global, Local, and Focal Mechanical Features of the Spinal Organ

This method of reasoning is clinically essential as it compartmentalizes the spine into global, local, and focal categories without losing sight of the congruency of the whole structure. This means that when we put our hands on one or two segments for investigation, we are able to see it in relation to its parts. As such, we can investigate the spine intelligently for related lesion patterns that could be affected. We know already that the spine is more than a collection of bones; it has influence on, and is affected by, all lines of force carried by all structures that lead to and from it, including the position of the head and limbs. Before explaining the influence of the external frame on the spine, it is worth prioritizing these three perspectives on the spine itself for reasons derived from pertinent clinical observations about neurophysiology.

Many times, especially with junior practitioners, their well-meaning efforts are driven to fix each and every lesion on the spine. They do not yet fully appreciate that they are dealing with living tissue that responds to their treatment. If there is an isolated area that needs treatment, the best course of action may (or may not) be to treat that area. The practitioner informed about the collective mechanics of the spine will be better able to palpate and direct the treatment necessary to aid the restoration of health in the individual. If we note lesions within spinal curves and we correct it with a global approach, not only does that inform us about the nature of the lesion with respect to mechanics, but it also provides us with a differential diagnosis if it does not correct. If this is the case, it means that we can now consider providing a more localized treatment within an arch. We might look for key lesions and holding patterns in and around the spine and/or look at how these three areas are affected by vectors of force—emerging from the compressive forces above and below—that buckle the curve.

If treatment has been administered in accordance with the above two concepts and the lesion persists, we can look more focally at the divisions between these three primary transition zones within the arch. As a cause or an effect, a subluxation of a segment or segments within a division could be owing to direct trauma and/or visceral lesioning. Again, it is important not to jump too quickly into treating those particular segments. We must remember to look to our mechanics and myology, and apply those principles to the anatomical position of the articular surfaces in question.

Global, Local, Focal Treatment of the Arch

We should continuously strive to treat from the same global, local, and focal principle. These self-healing and self-regulating processes are inherent in the collectivity of the body and its parts. From this perspective, it is impossible to treat the thoracic spine without considering the condition of cervical regions (and vice versa). Bringing the body back to its own collective, coordinated balance should be the desired goal. If we treat the majority of a curve in relation to its components, the health within adjacent curves will influence the discord among segments that are not coordinated within the arch where it resides. If influence can be observed, we know to look at the top, middle, and bottom of each arch, and then to the individual segments that lay between these areas, while contextualizing these observations within our differential diagnosis and palpation.

Introducing the Principle of Correlation 1.0

There are two ways of looking at the *principle of correlation* but only one that matters for our purposes. The first is by definition: to correlate something, osteopathically, means to put the parts of a thing back into order. The second way is a bit more complex because it addresses the *why* and *how* to put the parts where they belong. Without a clear methodology, it is easy for operators to lose focus. Without a way of looking at the body collectively, they are doomed to chase lesions without rhyme or reason. With the principle of correlation, however, we have a way of seeing how one lesion feeds another, and how we can reverse engineer our findings in the sequencing of our treatment. In the next section, we will show how to use this principle to help navigate the mechanics we have been working through.

Assisting versus Doing

This subsection continues with the principle of correlation, but elucidates it by explaining how we go from an orthopaedic understanding of the body to an osteopathic one. Under the first banner, we might look at the arm according to theoretical models of how the upper limb is supposed to function. We test it in relation to its joint mechanics and treat any restriction we find there. Similarly, if we are examining the thoracic spine, we palpate and look for a segment or group of segments that are following the typically opposite side coupling, and then we apply treatment to correct it. Not only is this approach labour-intensive, but it also treats the body in isolation; it does not relate the arm to the thoracic spine, nor the thoracic spine to the arm. More than this, it does not look to see how the arches of the spine, particularly the anterior arches, might be influencing either the arm or thoracic spine. This scenario will be detailed further, but we are hoping that the reader is already seeing the wisdom of addressing, via collective mechanics, those factors that could be influencing the two lesions. The guiding principle is, of course, that if we do not look, we do not find it. We must remember that our goal is to facilitate the propagation of health. We cannot enhance vitality without improving coordination. Coordination is only possible with an integrative approach that is allied with functional anatomy. Assessing and treating the body must mirror these ideals.

Conclusion

When we observe the spine, we consider the ankle, the position of the head, and/or the condition of the shoulder. We do not turn to orthopaedic testing (except in developing palpation skills in early operators). Instead, we rely on our knowledge of the mechanics, and from there, look for evidence of vitality or obstructions to it in the body. We then remove the obstructions according to the body's own laws. The assessment and treatment takes into account all forces acting upon it, and seeks to change structures in an integrative and sustainable way. This takes time, training, and discipline, but is ultimately achievable. The forces acting on the body, and the spine in particular, are abundant and profound; by correctly understanding what and how these forces may be influencing our mechanical ideal of the body, the opportunity for success in treatment is increased.

In this chapter, we covered the importance of mechanics as the ideal model for adjusting the dysfunctional anatomy back to its relatively normal position. We also discussed the principle of global, local, and focal as it pertains to investigating the spinal organ as a unit, as a group of arches, and as key points within each arch that express common lesioning. We ended the chapter by explaining the difference between orthopaedic and osteopathic treatment. In the next chapter, we analyze the influence of lesioning to and from the limbs. As we do this, we will dispel some theoretical models that might be in the reader's mind, bringing the mechanical back to the functional anatomy so that we can have a rational approach to mapping acute, chronic, and chronic/acute lesions with ascending or descending patterns.

2.7 The Limbs and Ascending/Descending Lesions

Clinical versus Theoretical Mechanical Models

In this chapter, we look more focally at the limbs and their influence on the polygonal mechanics. We have developed a practical model that can be used clinically. This is not always something that happens in osteopathy, despite the good intentions of other theoretical models of mechanics to help practitioners navigate the multitude of variances in the clinic room. These other models—when they are truly examined, practiced, and then questioned—are nothing more than guides. They might serve for academic exercises, but we would like our approach to be as practical as possible from the outset. That is why we have traced our collective mechanical model back to the functional anatomy rather than basing it on intangible theories that ignore Wolf's Law.

Theoretical Models of Spinal Mechanics

As much as possible, we depict an osteopathic model that focuses on the functional anatomy of each particular spine by offering frames of reference that are dictated by the anatomy. This is different than having a theoretical model address abstract lines where force should be traveling through. Such a model can be frustrating for practitioners, for no two functional spines are alike, let alone pathological spines. If practitioners fixate on these lines as the only way to help patients instead of returning function where function is lost, they will have a difficult time finding success in their clinical work.

Whenever there is a change in the angulation of facets, there is going to be a change in the function of gravity through those facets (and vice versa). More specifically, whenever there is a change in the force of gravity through a facet, there is also a change in the angulation of the facets responsible for distributing those forces that then affect physiological function. For example, as gravity travels down the C-spine, its first deviation is at the OA and then at the upper dorsals. We know that these areas, together with the middle of the arch, are of concern because of the changes that take place in the angulation of the facets, which are attempting to redistribute the forces from one curve to another. We can accept this synopsis to be true. We would never want to rely, however, on a model that says only C4 (because it is, by default, the middle of the arch and therefore deserving of our attention solely based on this fact) should be considered as the key segment in treatment, unless C4 was in lesion. Even then, as already mentioned, we are continually looking for the cause, not the result, that led to C4 being in lesion. Practitioners know well that Wolf's Law is always at play, and as such, the changes in the distribution of forces also changes the makeup of the skeletal system. Depending on the lesion's age, a dramatic transformation can occur in the angulation of the facets in and around these areas. This would mean that the centre for oscillation (if there is one) would be shunted to another section of the spine, therefore causing different probabilities for varying pathological vectors.

It is also naive to think that gravity is the only element responsible for altering the distribution of force through the spine, as there are somatic and organic lesions that could pull and twist the body into any number of positions. We also know that lesioning can be unilateral and/or bilateral, which further complicates the theory. As an example, we have the upper and lower girdles to address. Surely, the position of the upper girdle pulling with a unilateral declination would generate adverse tension on one part of the spine over another. This will influence not only the neurology to and from the spine, but also the trabeculation of the spine in relation to the demands placed on it by the soft tissue between the girdle and the spine.

We ask that practitioners always search out the functional mechanics when taking in abstract theories, and seek clinical proof in the application of these models.

Let Structure and Function Guide Us

To reiterate, the polygon model we propose is clinical in its application. Much of the assessment and treatment for this can be done on the coronal plane to address sidebending/rotation and torsional strains. As a result, it does not matter if the patient is restricted to being in seated, supine, prone, or lateral recumbent positions. We also know that if we are able to diagnose and treat a lesion on one plane, Nelson's Third Law reminds us that we will affect it on all planes. We have also stated that our model is based on the functional anatomy. The polygonal model itself mirrors the major muscle groups of the body, and takes into consideration their position, quality of mobility, and tissue texture in relation to the hard tissues of the body. These muscles are, then, used in both diagnosis, treatment, and reassessment. The limbs and their girdles are attachment sites for these major muscles, which means we can use the limbs as levers not only to assess but to treat the body simultaneously (our principle of integration in practice). As such, we are then able to treat both the symptom and the cause, for as one element in the chain links to another—either from the spine out, or from the limb into the spine—we are able to resolve both proximal and distal lesions with optimal impact. Let us now take a moment to explore how these points can be made clearer with a discussion of the upper and lower limbs.

Exploring Anatomy

We bring up practical versus theoretical models because we know how easy it is for practitioners to get lost in material that might be interesting to study but not altogether applicable in treatment. We seek a balance between the practical and the theoretical to ensure that instruction does not get in the way of learning. For example, when it comes to the lower limb, a practitioner must learn the ligaments, muscles, and neurovascular structures in and around the knee, but they must also see the knee as a whole just like an engineer would. While "like an engineer" is often a catchphrase in osteopathy, is it really understood? What is the perspective of the engineer versus the anatomist?

We continually invite practitioners to explore, investigate, and examine the anatomy with the notion that their questions should shape the way they understand the body as a collective unit of function. They should also consider the structures and attend to the *why* and *how* of the knee in terms of its construction. They should ask, "Why is it structured this way," and "What is that structure best at doing, and why is this so?" We can also use our principle of global, local, and focal by first looking at the long strap muscles that cross the knee down to the tibial plateau, and then to the ligaments that hold the joint together. In this way we build a realistic, functional understanding of all the contributing parts of the knee—and not just a simple lexicon of components listed in an anatomy book.

Let us consider the knee further. When we look at the plateau, we can see that it has a flat surface on a horizontal plane with grooves in the middle and on either end; this configuration simultaneously helps the joint bear weight and provides stability through its primary motions of flexion and extension. As we look closer at the ligaments, we can see which ones are larger and thicker and how they direct motion mechanics that could cause problems owing to twists, shears, and torsions from beneath or above. By pondering what the structure would be good at doing based on its design—including all the parts extending to and from it—practitioners can formulate a mental picture of a three-dimensional image of the body, one that is based on functionality rather than memorization of biological terms.

We invite the reader to pay close attention to the knee by asking these questions, and to then apply those same questions to every other structure in the human body. We should note the similarities and differences between structures while asking these questions: How does this structure support and abate motion and/or load travelling through it? How could that influence the structures above and below it? Why does the primary motion change from one structure to the next? How does the angulation of structures change from one area to another and why? What does that facilitate in the functional, vascular, neurological, lymphatic, endocrine, and organic fields that influence the health of the body?

Osteopathic versus Orthopaedic Mindsets

It is vital to establish this inquisitive mind in practitioners early on because it offers clues about the cause, *not* the effects, of the primary lesion. If they memorize lists rather than attempt to understand the body as a dynamic unit of function, they run the risk of seriouslymisreading Still and the early American osteopaths who are our Classical source on the science of osteopathy. Without this foundational perspective, there would be little difference in meaning between "orthopaedic" and "osteopathic." For instance, it is fine to say, "Find it,

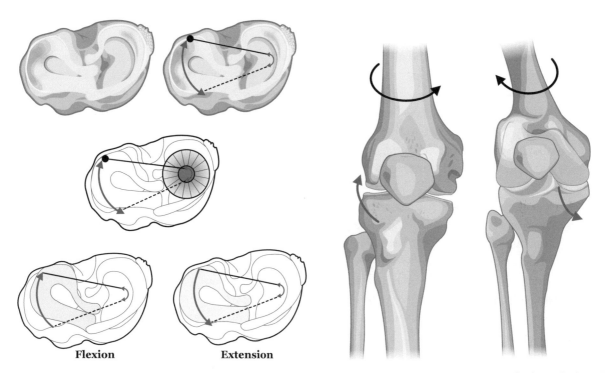

Flexion   **Extension**

In closed chain movement, the motion of the medial condyle of the femur is restricted by the thick medial collateral ligament, creating a pivot point upon the medial tibial plateau.

As the knee flexes and extends, the lateral condyle of the femur and the lateral meniscus shifts posterior and anterior upon the tibial plateau respectively.

Knee Extension: The lateral condyle of the femur reaches the physiological barrier while the medial condyle of the femur continues moving through its range of motion, creating posterolateral glide of the tibial plateau.

Knee Flexion: The lateral condyle of the femur reaches the physiological barrier while the medial condyle of the femur continues moving through its range of motion, creating anteromedial glide of the tibial plateau.

FIG. 27: The practitioner should look to the why and how of structures in terms of their construction. They should ask, "Why is it structured this way" and "What is that structure best at doing? And why is this so?"

fix it, and leave it alone," but what happens when we find a multitude of lesions? As our palpation skill improves, we notice more fibrosity here, a lack of motion there, all in areas that, prior to the increase in our skill level, we had not noticed lesioning beforehand. When that happens, how do we know what to treat? Without a way of working through the body collectively, operators will either be debilitated by their diagnostic findings or run around the table in a futile attempt to correct every lesion in the body. It also leaves them in a position where they are correcting without the principles of integration, and so the changes they do make are less likely to promote stability. For these reasons, we need to establish a difference between an orthopaedic understanding of the body and an applied osteopathic one. We need to know how to fix the proper areas, leave the body alone, then come back and fix the next series of lesions (and so on) with confidence and certainty.

Descending Lesions: The Lower Limb

When talking about the limbs, we should be thinking like engineers do about pulley systems, particularly the tension lines and the rotatory hubs between them. In the lower limb, the hubs are the innominates, and in the upper limb, the shoulder girdles. The two hubs are on opposing planes because of their respective responsibilities: the former are primarily for weight bearing and locomotion, which operates primarily on the sagittal plane; the latter is primarily on the coronal plane. Both are responsible for a number of different functions, including fluid mechanics: the lower limb pumps fluid back to D11/12 most efficiently via its sagittal mechanics, while the upper girdle uses its torsional vectors to distribute and receive blood and lymphatic fluid to and from the heart. The diaphragm sits on a transverse plane to mediate and coordinate the exchange of gas and fluids between these sagittal and coronal movements—to great effect. Knowing the prominent motion for each girdle is important, as our primary adjustment is always on their respective planes, and each of these planes needs to be coordinated with the others just mentioned. Our treatment is dictated by the functional anatomy and not by some arbitrary points to be memorized.

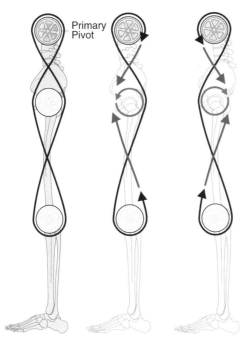

Primary Pivot

FIG. 28: If there is a shift in rotation of the innominate—either flexed or extended—the changes in the tension lines will then cause lesioning in the functioning of the lower limb, such as the knee.

In the lower limb, the anterior/posterior tension lines are the flexors and extensors of the lower limb that run off the central hub of the innominate, with the femoral head as its axis of rotation. Typically, there is a 60/40 split between the posterior and anterior tension lines; however, that balance is not possible if the innominate is sitting in the wrong

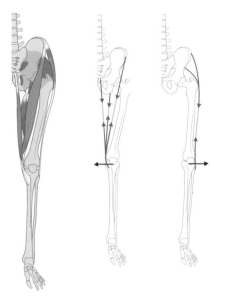

FIG. 29: This diagram shows how the altered axis (resulting from an innominate in the wrong position) will either cause a bilateral or unilateral shear (anterior or posterior) or torsion (internal or external) of the tibial plateau.

position. If there is a shift in rotation of the innominate—either flexed or extended—the changes in the tension lines will then cause lesioning in the functioning of the lower limb, such as the knee.

In this example informed by our functional anatomy, there are powerful muscles that hang off the innominate and attach to the inferior part of the lower limb. The altered axis, resulting from an innominate in the wrong position, will either cause torsion or a bilateral or unilateral shear—anterior or posterior, internal or external—of the tibial plateau. The next logical question must then be: What is the cause of this altered position?

Ascending/Descending Lesions 1.0

The lesion may be extending from above and/or below. On the one hand, we can reason that the malposition of the innominate can be greatly influenced from above by the lumbar spine. If the lumbars are loaded incorrectly, bi- or unilaterally, a bi- or unilateral pelvic tilt can result. This tilt is often evident in a compensating pattern where we find lumbar spine sidebending to the right and rotation to the left. Here, the right innominate will be anterior, and the left will be posterior, both of which affect the tension lines that descend to create a tibial torsion at the knee. This is where osteopathic adages, such as "The knee is not the knee," become palpable. We can see that there is a descending chain of cause and effect where the expression of the lesion is facilitated by the weakest link in that chain—that being, in this case, the knee (although it could be the ankle, or the bladder, or the upper T-line, for that matter). Exemplified here is a descending lesion pattern, where the lumbars influence the innominates that, in turn, influence the position of the knee. Practitioners take note: it is futile to treat the symptom of dysfunction for its own sake. Of course there are times when symptoms emanating from the knee must be alleviated, such as in acute cases, but only after we have addressed the root cause.

SB | Closed facets | Unilateral extension   Rotation | Open facets | Unilateral flexion

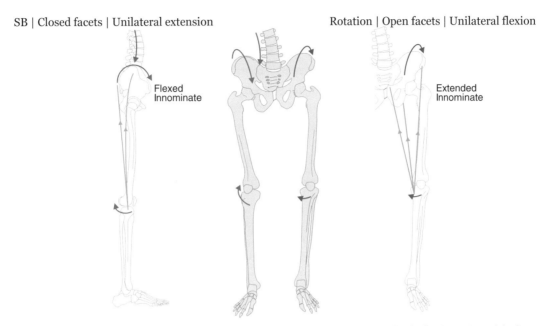

Flexed
Innominate

Extended
Innominate

FIG. 30: The malposition of the innominate can be greatly influenced from above by the lumbar spine. If the lumbars are loaded incorrectly, bi- or unilaterally, we can get bi- or unilateral pelvic tilt. Here we find the lumbar spine sidebending to the right and rotating towards the left. The right innominate will be anterior, and the left, posterior, affecting the tension lines that go down to create a tibial torsion at the knee.

Our scope, of course, does not terminate at the lumbar spine. We know that the lumbar spine is influenced by the upper T-line, which can often make the lower T-line oblique so that the hubs of the innominate are running in differing directions. Now the knee is being influenced by a long chain dysfunction—from the shoulder, to the hip, to the knee. This long chain can have mechanical influence down to the ankle and foot. If we then add the lower lesion at the talus, we have an even longer chain that implicates the entire body. Likewise, if the navicular and/or talus bones are not sitting in their correct position—owing to a high ankle sprain, for instance—torsion and/or shearing of the tibial plateau can result, which then impacts the tension lines that traverse the tibial plateaus and ascend to the innominates. In typical chain fashion, this then influences the position of lumbar spine, which alters the position of the upper T-line. Described here is an intricate example of an ascending lesion from the lower limb.

Ascending/Descending Lesions 2.0:
Chronic Acute Cycles of Lesioning

When considering the chain lesion expounded above, the necessity for global, local, and focal perspectives of the lesion picture becomes ever more apparent for diagnosis and treatment. Not only does it allow us to see how the body is working (or not working) collectively—as is the case with the knee lesion example—but it also provides a logical way to progress to the knee. This is why, in the end, we understand that unless the knee is injured due to direct trauma, this type of lesion is typically not a localized event. Our diagnosis and treatment should mirror this understanding. We must be able to see what is influencing the knee from above and below, and then identify how that chronic dysfunction contributes to other lesions (either somatic or organic, as the case may be).

If the knee can be described as "acute" resulting from a chronic hip or shoulder injury that is never corrected, it can feed back into the body to create, not a chain of dysfunction, but a cycle of lesioning. The now-chronic knee becomes a chronic back, which then further affects the shoulder line, and may then manifest as a liver problem due to the torsional forces from above and below that now shear parts of the liver field. The liver is never merely the liver, just as the shoulder is never merely the shoulder. When it's the shoulder, it's the lumbar spine, it's the knee, it's the hip, and so on.

Osteopathic Integrative Treatment

This ability to spiral logically in and out of an area is important for a number of different reasons. First, it provides constant reference points through which to measure the effectiveness of our treatment. Second, it also establishes an effective way of formulating a treatment plan that follows a logical sequence guided by the differentials assessed during treatment. Third, and most importantly, it follows the principle of integration where we are treating up and down the chain globally, locally, and/or focally when necessary. Therefore, we are never misguided about our next step in treatment, for when we find a localized lesion in one area, we look for compensation, and, within that compensation, move up and/or down the chain to break the cycle of lesioning. This process will be elucidated in Section III in our discussion of the difference between primary, secondary, and tertiary lesions. With this knowledge, we will then have a way to prioritize the lesion pattern(s), which will give us the best protocol for treatment.

The Upper Limb

We have already begun discussion of the upper limb by noting the scapulae as hubs on a coronal plane with tension lines going to the spine and upper limbs (both dorsally and ventrally). We have also noted that its pathological vectors can have great influence on the lower girdle. As such, we do not want to simply reiterate what was mentioned with respect to the lower limb and vice versa. Nor do we want the discussion to turn into an orthopaedic explanation of the structures that comprise the upper girdle and limb. Instead, by drawing on the above literature to formulate an osteopathic understanding of the lower limb, the reader should already be thinking about the similarities and differences between the two structures. We should be considering the similarities and differences between the knee and elbow, asking, "Why are they different? What are they best at doing? How is movement controlled and facilitated and for what reasons?" In addition, the student practitioner should also be thinking of how the structure of the upper girdle intersects with our exposition of polygon mechanics.

Planes of Function Governed by Structure

The scapulae are the innominates of the upper girdle. They are large, boney structures with large strap muscles that aid in the mobility and motility of the upper limb and thorax. Different than the innominates of the pelvis, the scapulae are on the coronal plane. This allows them to accommodate the primary motion mechanics of the thoracic spine, sidebending/rotation, while providing a stable foundation for the upper limb to move along a perpendicular plane of motion sagittally. This sagittal plane motion of flexion/extension becomes more prominent as we move further from the spine to become a powerful pump for proper fluid and lymphatic dynamics.

The clavicles and scapulae work together to help stabilize the upper limb. When the former are in their correct position, they help wedge the latter apart, directing them down and out. The result is two-fold: first, the scapulo-thoracic (ST) joint is able to coordinate the weight of the arm in a neutral position during ambulation; second, the rotator cuff muscles are better able to mobilize the arm through flexion/extension up to about ninety degrees of abduction. Consequently—and as a rule—if there is a problem with motion up to about 90 degrees, we typically have a problem with the gleno-humeral (GH) joint. After that, we should examine the condition of the scapula-thoracic joint and its ability to glide along the thoracic wall to permit motions overhead. This information should help practitioners in assessing the upper limb in relation to the head, neck and thorax. Practitioners at this point should ensure that the spine is in order, that the upper and lower polygons are stacked on top of one another correctly, that the ribs are in their correct position to permit the internal/external rotation of the scapulae along the thoracic wall, and that the soft tissues of the scapulo-thoracic joint are situated appropriately. In addition, it is important to consider neurologically the condition of the cervical spine in relation to the upper limbs and how they are interacting with the upper and lower polygons.

Ascending/Descending Lesions 3.0:
Exploring the Functional Anatomy as Systems

There are other factors that could be affecting the upper girdle other than those mentioned above (and we have already discussed many of them, in one form or another). That said, it is worth considering how the augmentation of functional anatomy leads to poor respiration of tissues throughout the body, which can create any number of pathologies. Clinically, we note that when there is apposite GH and ST rhythm, there are fewer problems on the vascular end, which includes the function of the lymphatics. If the shoulders are fibrosed, however, they will be pinned down on the thoracic cage. The mirrored motion that should be allowed on the coronal plane between the scapulae and the thoracic cage abates clavicular and rib motion during the inhalation and exhalation phases. Without full respiration, the lungs cannot feed oxygen to all the cells of the body via the blood. If we return to our quadrant theory, we know the upper and lower girdle are mediated at D11/12, the primary pivot, the mediator of the subcostal epigastric fossa and the solar plexus. Without proper motion in the shoulder, the hip will also shift to compensate. At this point, we have a number of neurological and lymphatic factors that need consideration.

Distally, we can see how the body's ability to shunt the waste products via the lymphatics would also be compromised. The folds along the axial line are large central locations for lymph nodes. The ambulation of the limbs, together with the movement of the thorax during the respiration cycle, mechanically aid the quality of gas exchange and lymphatic supply and distribution. Again, going back to our quadrant theory, we can see how a restricted shoulder on one side of the body, and a restricted hip on the other, can compromise the lymphatics.

Ascending and Descending Lesions 4.0: Another Perspective

We usually think of treating limbs when acute; however, if left unattended for any period of time, these acute conditions can influence any number of structures, including the visceral field. We usually liken this scenario to having a rock in a shoe. At the end of the day, the foot is not the only thing that is sore, as the whole body feels the effects of having to ambulate around that foreign pivot, which changes the functional mechanics of the entire body. This can happen, as we have described, via discord between D11/12 as a result of an unlevelling of the T-lines. Yet we must also consider the possible influence of a distal, or ascending, lesion from the upper limb to the cervical spine by way of the brachial and cervical plexus, which then has influence on the organic field below.

In this way, an issue with the arm can have an ascending lesion originating from the periphery and entering the central axis (the spine). As the carrying angle irritates the central axis, the heart and lung field might also be irritated, both mechanically and neurovascularly. In this instance, if the limb is anterior and internally rotated, it will produce strain through the posterior line and into the heart and lung field. The autonomic distribution for these organs thus becomes affected by the mechanical lesion; however, because the arm is forward to the hip, it creates a long diagonal axis, which then has every opportunity to irritate even the digestive and gastric fields.

Conclusion

There are many ways of addressing a long chain lesion complex, but as we have stressed throughout this work, the mechanics offer an ideal foundation from which to discover the actual cause of dysfunction. Again, this does not mean that the correction will happen right away; it does mean, nonetheless, that the correction can come sooner, and in a way that gives more of a chance for the body to accept the guidance of the practitioner in aiding the restoration of health. Let's now move from a simple mechanical understanding that facilitates diagnosis and consider the application of treatment. With application in mind, we will look to the mechanical influence of the thorax.

2.8 The Thorax

Review of Collective Mechanics

At this point, we have created a layered presentation of our collective mechanics in a logical, progressive way. First, we introduced the quadrants and explained how the organs and their neurovascular pathways need their own respective spaces to function correctly. Then we introduced our polygon mechanics that show how soft tissue lines running to and from the limbs—as well as hard tissues running along the central axis, augmenting each quadrant— affect how well the compromised organs and neurovasculature are able to function within patterns of compensation. From there, we introduced different types of lesioning within the polygon structure, including key lesions and secondary holding patterns that interfere with the natural ambulation cycle and collective symmetry (rhythm) of the body. We then applied this understanding to discuss how, by examining ascending and descending lesions that affect the optimal function of somatic and organic fields, the limbs can influence these key lesions and their holding patterns. We also have tried to frame all of these patterns within the principle of correlation so that we can better diagnose the cause of lesioning rather than focus on the resultant forces that culminate in the expression of dysfunction. For example, we explained how the spine is a series of arches that influence one another in a dynamic way. At this point, we must add another layer to our mechanical understanding through consideration of the thorax. First, we will explain the *what*, then we will discuss the *why*.

Six Divisions

When it comes to the thorax, practitioners have an easy time making the subject more complicated than it needs to be. They get caught up in trying to determine sidebending and rotation patterns and flexion/extension lesions that might not really be there. While the body's ability to compensate is compromised, the reflex may not be fully engaged and, therefore, there might not be a full-blown osteopathic lesion. This illustrates why our overall discussion has gone from the outside to the inside, using global, local, and focal as our principle for determining the correct level of lesioning. Our goal is to provide a course of treatment that is the least invasive and the most effective. As we have noted, the holding patterns of one lesion can often have an influence on other areas of facilitation that are not relevant until each layer is resolved, one layer at a time. This is how we progress logically through the body and read and react to what we find—layer by layer—to expose the key lesion(s) and restore health. Let's now look at an example of how this might be done.

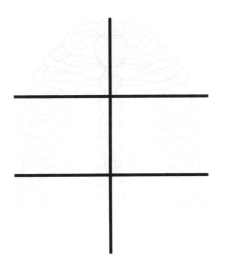

FIG. 31: The thorax divided into six section: the upper ribs, middle and lower ribs on the right and left sides of the thorax.

If the holding patterns of key lesions persist, particularly after clearing the long lines that feed into them, then the lesioning must be deeper. This scenario demands that we look more locally, particularly at the thorax, as there is an abundance of physiological centres routing from the spine that affect both the organic and somatic fields. Therefore, having a logical way of proceeding through the thorax, without getting lost in the minutiae of what the spine and ribs might be doing, is essential. To aid this process, we have divided the thorax into six sections. The four quadrants are still relevant to our model of reasoning with the only difference being that we are looking more locally. Rather than view the thorax as quadrants, we divide the thorax into thirds horizontally, according to rib function. The first horizontal division includes the upper ribs; the second, the mid ribs; and third, the lower ribs. We then separate these horizontal lines with a vertical line down the centre, dividing the thoracic cage into right and left along the spine dorsally, and the sternum and linea alba ventrally.

With these divisions now in place, we are better able to see patterns of lesioning that we can then categorize into what we call *slope* and *pitch*. The direction of the slope of the thorax has to do with sidebending and rotation. The pitch, or angulation of the thorax, corresponds to flexion/extension of the pelvis. Clinically, we will commonly note changes in slope and pitch between left and right, and between the upper, middle, and lower divisions. This helps when assessing whether there are compensating or non-compensating patterns, as well as determining the physiological effects of lesioning through this area.

Other Models

Already, readers should see that we are proposing a much more sophisticated way for assessing the thorax while considering the relevance of rib positioning. Conventional understanding of rib mechanics typically focuses on the ventral surface and whether or not the ribs are

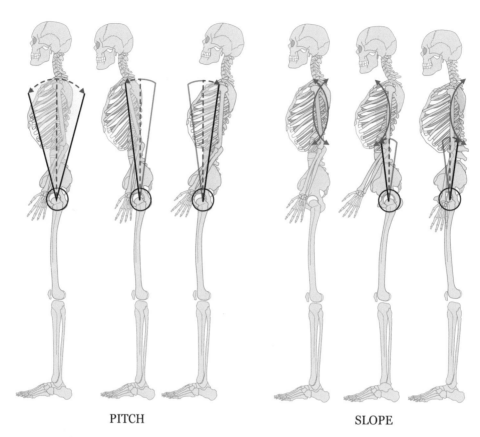

PITCH   SLOPE

FIG. 32: The direction of the slope of the thorax has to do with sidebending and rotation. The pitch, or angulation, of the thorax corresponds to flexion/extension of the pelvis.

inhaled (up) or exhaled (down). The standard method of correction first considers the spine in order to improve neurovascular innervation to the somatic and organic fields, which could be influencing the position of the rib. However, we must not forget that the ribs, as much as the spine, are expressions of the internal environment, be they the cause or result of lesioning on either field of influence. If we have defined the external frame as the limbs and polygons, and the internal frame as the motor line, then this internal environment of the throat (within the visceral field) is the innermost frame. The case for this determination requires some explanation, particularly with reference to the functional anatomy of the thoracic cage.

We use this language of "frames" because they follow lines of tension that form geometrical patterns that are palpable. If we step back and view the trapezius muscle again, we see that it is forming a triangular frame bridged between the boney structures. As we recognize this normal triangular pattern, it is easier to identify the abnormal or, more specifically, the distortion in the lines of pull. This means we are able to infer a change in that frame and the frames relating to it. In other words, this provides an alternative way of conceptualizing a layer-by-layer, tissue-by-tissue approach to diagnostics. Although we do not base our diagnosis on the soft tissue alone, it will either follow or oppose the other frames we are discussing. Noting an abnormality on the surface tissue expedites the exploratory process in treatment.

Three Purposes

The thoracic cage has three functions that we are interested in discussing: support, protection, and attachment. These three are interrelated, of course, and should be thought of as such, but of greater importance is how they impact our ability to correctly assess and treat the slope and pitch of the region in question. We know that the cage is a resilient structure that protects the internal environment from the external (and vice versa). If the slope and pitch are correct, there is enough space for the full expansion of the lung during inspiration, and for contraction of the ligaments surrounding the anterior and posterior attachments of the ribs during expiration. The unabated rhythm of this mechanism has neurovascular influence on every level. Structurally, it also supports the arch mechanics previously introduced. The ribs, together with the shoulder girdle, help neutralize forces of influence from the anterior curves.

Support and attachment are very closely related and are quite important as we begin to recognize the correlation between the soma and the organic fields. Through assessment of pitch and slope, we can use our mechanical diagnosis regarding the presentation of thoracic hard and soft tissues, for example, as an expression of further lesioning in the lung field.

The Three Divisions of the Ribs

As already stated, the ribs are divided into three horizontal sections—upper, middle, and lower—each with their own influences on and from the organic field via the autonomic nervous system. They are divided according to their mechanical functions, as will be discussed later in the chapter, but first we consider their organic influence. In the first division, we are concerned with the upper ribs as they affect the heart and lungs. Distally, we are also interested in brachial neuralgia—but that is not our current focus. The heart and lung field has everything to do with fluid distribution and supply via the blood, which, subsequently, determines its toxicity by means of gas exchange. We are still concerned with heart and lung dynamics in the middle division, but we are also thinking about digestive breakdown and assimilation of fuel via the upper gastrointestinal tract (including stomach, pancreas, liver, and gall bladder). In the lower division, we are concerned with the inferior portion of the gastrointestinal tract and execratory functions.

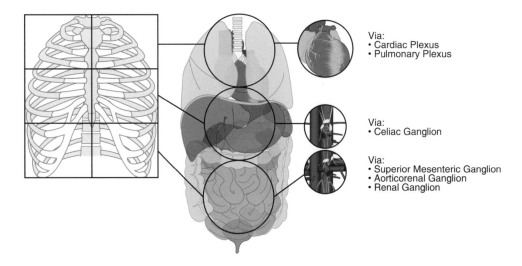

Via:
• Cardiac Plexus
• Pulmonary Plexus

Via:
• Celiac Ganglion

Via:
• Superior Mesenteric Ganglion
• Aorticorenal Ganglion
• Renal Ganglion

FIG. 33: A look at the organic influence of the ribs through the nervous system.

Pair Organ Theory

If we pay close attention to these divisions and the responsibility of the organs in each, we notice a pairing of organ functions. In the first division, we see heart and lung; in the second, stomach and liver; in the third, kidney and bladder and small and large intestines. From here, we are able to ascertain the degree of lesioning being expressed throughout the body with our assessment of pitch and slope. If the lesioning is contained to a paired organ system, it is considered a chain lesion. If the lesioning includes another pairing, it is considered a complex chain. All lesions will be a combination of at least one complex chain, but we must also consider the degrees of lesioning, whether they are ascending or descending, and/or proximal or distal.

It should now be apparent how a change in pitch and slope can affect the organic field, either mechanically or physiologically. That said, it should always be remembered that a physiological influence is reflected in the anatomy of the rib and the structures attached to it. When we consider the autonomic distribution of sympathetic chain ganglia coming from the spine,

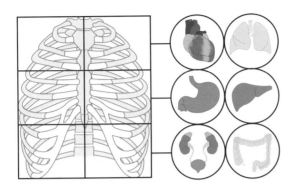

FIG. 34: Observing the rib divisions and the responsibility of the organs associated with each, we notice a pairing of organ functions. In the first division, we see heart and lung; in the second, stomach and liver; in the third, kidney and bladder and small and large intestines.

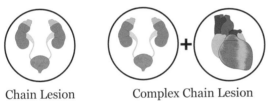

Chain Lesion   Complex Chain Lesion

FIG. 35: *Chain Lesion & Complex Chain Lesion.*

we should not just think of the direct innervation to its respective organs, but rather of its motor distribution on the neurovascular end.

We know that the motor nerve has a direct effect on the vasomotion of a vessel. Motor nerves in and around the autonomics have a role as both vaso-dilators and vasoconstrictors for the vascular system that supplies an organ. The motor nerve also figures heavily in the regulation of glandular secretions for digestion and assimilation. This is important to us osteopathically, for the motor reflex is what allows us to diag-nose the body from the outside through our palpation of the intrinsic muscula-ture of the spine (as well as the periph-eral musculature and the position of the rib). That same motor control has a re-flex arc in the erector mass and the soft tissues that attach to the spine and the surface of the rib. With that being the case, should we address the mechanical lesion of slope and pitch, we will influence the nerve force along the soft tissues of the rib and the spine; this will initiate a reflex arc on the organic field and the neurovascular systems that support it physiologically and mechanically.

Thoracic Strain Patterns

We know that the thoracic spine can be influenced from above and below by the position of the cervical and lumbar curves. As we stated in our explanation of the three functions of the rib, we also know that the thoracic cage aids in the support of dissipating force from each of these curves. That said, we have not yet indicated how to use this knowledge clinically. To flesh out the clinical picture, we will discuss a thoracic strain pattern.

We do this by integrating the "pair organ theory" with the three divisions of the ribs, in which case the thorax is divided into six sections. Again, there are the functional groupings of the upper ribs, the middle ribs, and the lower ribs, which are bisected by the motor line. Within these six divisions, there are certain patterns practitioners can expect to see from either the global compensation pattern or local compensation pattern of the thorax. For example, there could be an alternating triangular compensation pattern where there is flexion in the upper thorax on the left, middle thorax on the right, and lower thorax on the left. There can also be a bilateral compensation pattern, wherein the upper thorax is flexed, the middle thorax is extended, and the lower thorax is flexed. Of course, these are only examples; the body is capable of any variation, including flexion in the upper and middle to the left and lower right divisions, or a common sweep where there is unilateral flexion to one side or another.

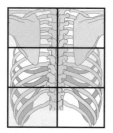 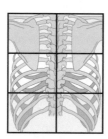 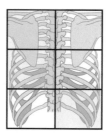 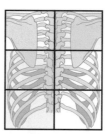 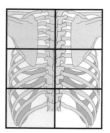

Example 1:
Unilateral Pattern
• Flexion upper left thorax
• Flexion middle right thorax
• Flexion lower left thorax

Example 2:
Bilateral Pattern
• Flexion upper thorax
• Extension middle thorax
• Flexion lower thorax

Example 3:
Other Patterns
• Flexion upper left thorax
• Flexion middle left thorax
• Flexion lower right thorax

Example 4:
Other Patterns
• Flexion upper right thorax
• Flexion middle left thorax
• Flexion lower left thorax

Example 5:
Other Patterns
• Flexion upper left thorax
• Flexion middle left thorax
• Flexion lower left thorax

FIG. 36: *Compensation within the six divisions.* Flexion is shown in blue.

After noting a combination of the pattern(s) above, practitioners can ascertain how their palpation for thoracic lesions does not just follow flexion/extension patterns, but also compensates for one another based on mobility. Indeed, it is common for practitioners to mistake a lack of motion or symmetry when palpating ribs, when in fact they are palpating the top of a strain pattern that is coming from either the spinal arches, the mycological field, or the visceral field. If they feel a group of ribs that are hard and without movement in one division, they might note that the ribs below can be exceptionally mobile. That mobility can occur on any axis, on any plane. The point between the immobility and mobility is the key lesion that the body begins to hinge around, forming its own compensation pattern with consequent secondary lesion patterns. These breaks often occur between the three divisions we have previously outlined and are typically painful to the touch. Using the six divisions helps compartmentalize the practitioner's diagnostics to identify these key lesions more quickly and effectively.

Let's consider in more detail an example of a bilateral compensation pattern in the thorax. If a patient presents with excess weight and has an exaggerated lumbar extension, the visceral field will be driven ventrally. This will increase tension on the diaphragm, which will increase the costal tension, right and left, along its sternal attachments, and centrally along the linea alba. The lower ribs will be caught in exhalation and the mid ribs will be pulled ventrally. However, to prevent the middle of the arch and its ribs from going into complete extension, the shoulder girdle pulls back against this force, which creates a break in the upper four ribs that then appear to be contracted (inhaled). That attempt to balance the thorax can then direct the head backward as the cervical spine attempts to mirror the lumbar spine and balance the tension from the compensated position of the upper girdles. We now have a cascade of events that will lead to a plethora of potential pathological conditions.

The poor function of the diaphragm produces problems with the stroke volume and vacuum of the respiratory cycle, which consequently alters the quality of the gas exchange. A hyper-sympathetic state then pervades the thoracic spine as the ribs are unable to spring back after inspiration, which means the tension does not drop off at the end of the breath cycle. As a result of this ventral drift, there is also strain placed on the linea alba. The strain pattern also translates to a stretch on the lung pleura, which is expressed in the intercostal tissues, which in turn restricts the flow of blood coming from the thoracic area into the abdominal area, which then can affect the vasomotion in the vessels to the stomach and upper GI. That change in regularity of flow could prevent blood from leaving the area, creating congestion and fermentation, which then sends toxic materials to the liver via the portal system. This compromises the packaging of the blood in the liver for combustion because the vasoconstriction also affects glandular secretions necessary for the up-building qualities of blood, degrading the entire constitution of the body. This hyper-sympathetic state, exacerbated by the ventral pull on the organ field, negatively affects the SI joints—particularly the left—leading to poor excretion. Now the liver is also being compromised by the small intestines and a whole host of spin-off effects; this potentially triggers the fluid processes of the kidney and bladder as they attempt to neutralize the toxic event manifesting in the body.

At this point, it seems futile to argue that the liver is just the liver or that the rib is just the rib. As with the lines of force affecting the polygons, the ribs and dorsal spine need to be integrated with a correlative methodology for correction. This correlative method can reverse these complex chain lesions that traverse paired lesion fields and create numerous problems for patients and practitioners alike. The above description serves as one possible example of a toxic event leading to a pathological manifestation of one disease process or another. Practitioners should consider other possibilities, as these strain patterns can also present themselves with fixation lesions in the lumbars and any myriad of variations extending from the somatic to the organic, and from the external to the internal frame.

Conclusion

With all this material on collective mechanics covered, practitioners should now be able to integrate its many levels into a workable, seamless model for applying osteopathic methods of diagnosis and treatment. We will further assist with these tasks in the next section of the book as we look at highlighting different perspectives on treatment approaches.

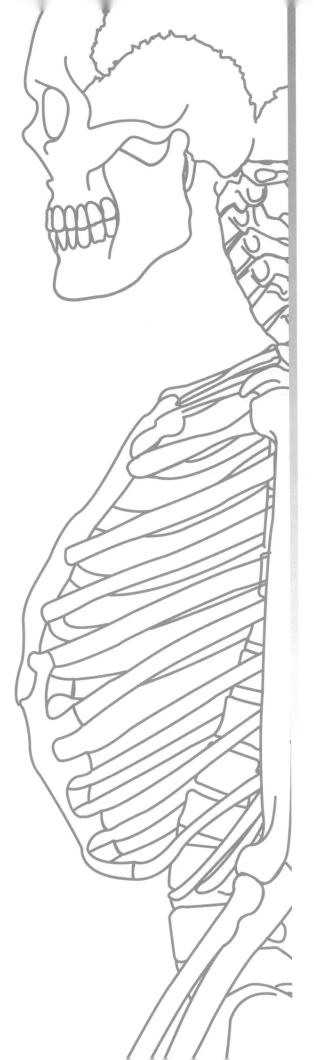

Section III:

Thoughts on Treatment

--------------------------------- SECTION III ---------------------------------

Thoughts on Treatment

3.1 Application of Collective Mechanics

The Application of Collective Mechanics in Treatment

Knowing the applications of collective mechanics in treatment is important to understand what practitioners palpate. Indeed, when we see mechanical stresses and strains between the upper and lower T-lines, the quadrants, and the polygons, we provide a three-dimensional matrix of the lesion from a palpatory perspective. All of these models are ways of understanding our diagnostic findings. Rarely, if ever, does a lesion in one area stay in that area. For instance, a lesion in the pelvis almost always has a knock-on effect on other areas of the body. This knock-on effect could be found in the visceral field, the shoulder, the upper limb, and/or the neck. Without a context for being able to anticipate, palpate, and interpret these findings, the intention of a practitioner is irrelevant.

When the theory and the palpation comes together, however, we have the ability to prioritize the primary, secondary, and tertiary lesions in ways that show their interrelationships with one another. For example, it is one thing to recognize a problem with the knee, the ribs, and/ or the right lung; it is another to correlate and bridge these lesions together—from the mechanical to the anatomical to the physiological—in ways that make sense clinically. Otherwise we are left only knowing that we have three areas in lesion without ever really understanding *why*. We know from Still that the study of anatomy for the sake of anatomy is a dead end. We must have a contextual framework for our practice, and this is where collective mechanics infuses anatomy with a meaning greater than the sum of its parts. Therefore, our goal from the beginning has been to bridge the disciplines constituting our practice in a way that allows us to converse with the body and promote its healthy functioning.

Under the banner of collective mechanics, practitioners will note there is an understanding of collective anatomy, collective physiology, and collective pathophysiology. All of these are reflected in the principle that the body is a dynamic unit of function. Therefore, our means of assessing is dynamic, focused on the body's unity and functionality. From there, we search for what needs to be done, all based on how we understand our palpation. So when a patient comes into the office with lower back pain, we are able to question, palpate, and deduce a host of related symptoms that could be at play.

Collective Mechanics and Stabilization

Imagine, for a moment, every frame referenced thus far as a separate piece of paper scattered on a desk. There is a piece of paper representing the fascial, the muscular, the boney, the neurovascular, the lymphatics, and visceral categories. As we assess and palpate with collective mechanics in mind, we are able to work through each of these pieces of paper, layer by layer, and adjust each one in relation to the others until we have a neat pile. That neat stack, where everything is in order, has better collective function in terms of organization. By knowing each of these layers, our palpation directly informs our treatment to bring these constituents into order. If practitioners can only feel one layer or another, they run the risk of failing to stabilize the body, and thereby risk a patient's pathology persisting or even metastasizing elsewhere. By knowing each layer, however, two things happen: practitioners become complete, dynamic osteopaths who do not favour one approach over another; and two, their patients have a greater likelihood of stabilizing after treatment, mechanically and physiologically.

Global, Local, and Focal Together with Primary, Secondary, and Tertiary

The concept of global, local, and focal dovetails with discussions of collective mechanics. The focalized lesion is not independent of the general pattern, and so by knowing more about the general pattern, we are then able to identify the focal pattern. As lesioning is a dynamic expression of dysfunction (and not a static issue), taking care of the general pattern often helps stem the cascading effects of the collective lesion pattern. When we are able to logically spiral through these three perspectives, the treatment for one part will have influence on and affect all others.

Let's look at our placatory diagnostics through collective mechanics using an example of a common lesion pattern. In this case, the patient with limited movement presents an acute L5/S1 lesion that is extremely painful. This lesion has an effect up the chain to D11/12, which is sore but not as painful or limited in motion as L5/S1. Together these two lesions ascend and create an anterior positioning of the left shoulder. The movement is slightly affected in this area, and there is little pain relative to the other two lesions. Should we focus on the baseline at L5/S1 and the primary pivot at L5/S1 while ignoring the asymmetrical swing from that shoulder, the patient's symptoms may improve temporarily but then recur a few weeks later. This is because the full lesion pattern was not identified and treated as part of our global, local, and focal perspective, which would have shown that the specific lesion at L5/S1 is primary, the primary pivot is the secondary lesion, and the shoulder is the tertiary lesion. The shoulder will continue to have an effect on the secondary and primary lesions, locally and focally, until it is cleared.

Why We Do Not Speak About Technique

In reviewing all of Still's works, there is a rather conspicuous de-emphasis of notions surrounding *technique*. He suggests, instead, that there are many different ways of administering treatment and that practitioners should figure out what works best for them. Why would he make this claim? More importantly, if we are following Still's advice, why would we put this kind of a book together? First of all, this is not a book about technique, but about processes based on, as he suggested, an understanding of the anatomy that requires us to use reason and logic. By employing differential diagnosis we do not, as Still writes, become engine wipers (essentially, low-ranking cleaners of dirt and soot from machinery). An appreciation of the collective mechanics renders us complete osteopaths who can understand the structure in its entirety.

If we were to focus on technique, however, there is a danger that practitioners will see treatment as something fragmented. From this perspective, the application of technique is carried out as a series of manipulations from one area of the body to another, not as something based on a dynamic understanding of how the lesion and pathology communicate through our palpation over increments of time. That dynamic understanding fosters the ability to move with the tissue in such a way as to render what could then be considered osteopathic "technique." Yet this technique—if we can qualify it that way—includes within its application a comprehensive understanding of the lesion in relation to its collective mechanics. There are many practitioners who have poor treatments but outstanding technique, simply because they are not dynamic in their thinking.

When Still suggests that no two general treatments are ever the same, he was not being facetious. He never used a "general treatment" as we know it because he recognized the mechanics' relationship to anatomy and physiology, and read and reacted to his palpation. This means that if someone were to receive two treatments, each would be fundamentally different. From Still's approach we learn that, if we are reading and reacting to the tissue in real time while conscious of the roles and responsibilities within the entire structure, we have a way of working *with* the body rather than making a series of manipulations *to* it.

3.2 Mechanics in Diagnosis and Treatment

Hands and Mind Working Together

Treatment is based on a diagnostic evaluation of the mechanical, anatomical, and physiological qualities of a lesion. One's approach has to be intelligent to see the patterns presented, and the message the lesion patterns provide. If practitioners are completely focused on the approach to treatment, they will not be thinking of what they are perceiving with their hands during assessment. The hands and brain must work together through the different frames of collective mechanics (as discussed in Section II) to understand the lesion and treat it correctly. We must be like master carpenters using implements of the trade: they do not necessarily think about their tools, as a lathe and hammer just as well become extensions of the body. They use these supplemental appendages with confidence and ease as they hold the blueprint of their work in their mind's eye.

It is easy to rely on a model such as the general treatment. If that routine does not fit the reality of the lesion, however, both operators and patients suffer. That is why we have taken—and will continue to take—so much time discussing the mechanics based on the anatomy of the patient that walks through the door, and not on a theoretical patient that exists in a textbook. That is also why there are no techniques discussed in this book. Instead, we will continue to focus on the mechanics, the anatomy, the physiology, and the pathophysiology that can be correlated with our findings to then establish a scientific method of deduction for working through the body. To this end, we are providing an algorithm more so than a routine, offering practitioners a model for clinically validated results.

Theory of Compensation and Polygonal Mechanics

While we have already attributed the theory of compensation to G. Zink, D.O., we should also note that his ideas of compensation are often misunderstood as only dealing with fascia. This was not his intent, and neither is it ours. Instead, we recognize the fascia as one of the tissues that can influence the body's ability to reconstitute balance, symmetry, and health for optimal function. If we understand compensation as part of the body's self-healing and self-regulating mechanisms, we can deploy it to assess the vitality of the patient by observing how well the body is compensating (or not), and how that compensation is affecting all tissues. We learn the most from this model when we integrate it with our polygonal mechanics.

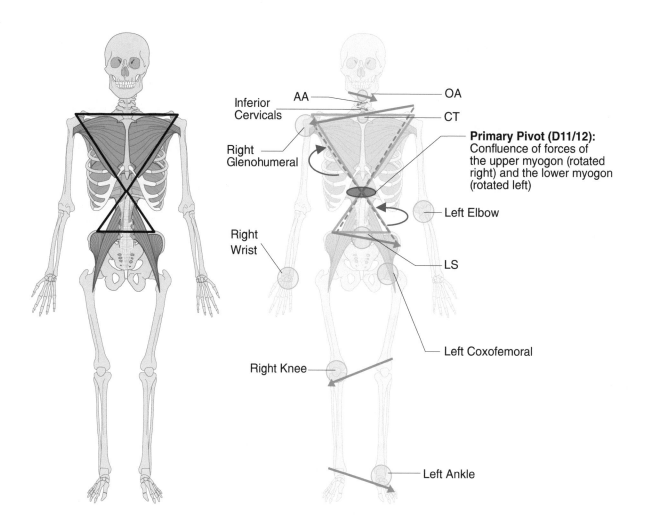

FIG. 37: *Theory of Compensation and Polygonal Mechanics.* Here we see Zink's Common Compensation Pattern overlaying polygonal mechanics in order to demonstrate the relationship between the two concepts.

By combining these two concepts, practitioners can better read the body as they reinforce the principle of identifying the normal from abnormal. If we know and expect a compensated pattern, anything that is found outside of that compensating framework should lead us down a path of further exploration. Herein lies the science of association in osteopathy: looking at the anatomical relationships between structures or, as we stated earlier in our discussion on the barrier, the pathways between structures. Significant in this mechanical model are structures that are observable and palpable to practitioners, which means the results both before and after treatment are also measurable. The burden of abstraction is alleviated as operators have a concrete model from which they may reason their way through treatments in logical, progressive ways.

From the Normal on the Coronal Plane

If the last section was about the *why* behind polygonal mechanics, this chapter is about the *what*. It is a blueprint of what we should expect to find in our observations—regardless of the patient's position—that can then be further explored with the patient in passive motion testing to determine the primary and secondary lesion patterns. Of course there are exceptions within this model, but let's be clear: if we do not define our intended outcome as restoring health to *normal*, we have nothing to which *abnormal* can be compared. We are, after all, working toward a standard of health, just as there are standards to writing, engineering, or the practice of law.

We will begin with a global look at the vertical line and the two T-lines. In our common compensated model of collective mechanics, readers will note a declination on the right upper T-line due to a right rotation in the thorax that is compensating for a left rotation around the primary pivot of D11/12, resulting in a declination to the left in the lower T-line. Before practitioners put their hands on a patient, they are anticipating what is normal in the region. This takes into account the CT, the TL, and the LS junctions and our central belt theory, offering a snapshot of what is happening at the major transition zones we have already discussed. Owing to their change from one motion potential to another, we can palpate and motion test (as areas of interest) each of the girdles and transition zones. In motion testing these areas, practitioners will also note the level of lesioned tissue from superficial to deep. This is significant, as it affords operators the choice of the best tool for treating the lesioned area: direct, indirect, and/or balance. Remember that this is only a global view and that we should take this common pattern further.

In looking more locally at the lumbar spine and pelvis, particularly on the coronal plane, there are compensations at play regardless of whether there is an ascending or descending pattern driving the lesion (within the general sidebend right, rotation left diagnosis). Many times, the lumbar sidebend is carried through to the sacrum, which is where we find the right pole anterior. Within this transition, however, it can be common for L5 to compensate for this general sweep and for sidebend/rotation in the opposite direction. This sidebend/rotation occurs because the iliolumbar ligament attached to the sacrum, the innominate, and L4/5 has great influence on the position of these structures; essentially, their tethering keeps these structures moving in the same direction. In either case, it is worth investigating and matching palpation with possible pathologies that relate to the autonomic distribution in the area.

This general sidebend of the lumbars is also reflected in the position of the innominates, where patients present with an anterior right, posterior left position that mirrors the side-bend, or anterior right position of the right transverse processes of the lumbar spine, and the posterior, or rotated, left transverse processes. If during palpation and motion testing practi-tioners find something different, they need to pause and consider what structures related to these could be influencing them and what their neuroendocrine consequences could be.

In transition from the base of the lower polygon to its apex, the primary pivot at D11/12 is typically rotated left, sweeping down to the innominates, which we find on the right following the sidebend into an anterior position, and on the left following the rotation into a posterior position. These rotatory lesions can generally be influenced by the soft tissue lines that con-nect to them, as well as the organ fields that are innervated by the lumbar splanchnic nerves and blood supply. With respect to the thoracic cage, if we remember our six divisions, we can typically see a thoracic strain pattern following the three horizontal divisions where the lower and upper right are rotated to the right and the middle division is rotated left. It would be prudent for practitioners to consider any influences from the organic tissues beneath the cage, as well as the tethering of the upper limbs in relation to the thorax.

As we transition to the cervical spine, we typically find a sidebend/rotation to the left in the lower cervical unit. Keep in mind, however, that the vertebrae close to the CT junction may mimic characteristics of the upper dorsal spine (and vice versa), in which case extra attention should be paid to how the structures in this area move in relation to their expected motion po-tentials and their compensatory capacity (given the overall lesion pattern). The compensation of the cervical spine is mirrored within the different parts of the upper complex, where the AA is typically rotated to the right, and the OA is sidebent left, rotated right.

With respect to the limbs, we would look for the compensation pattern to continue where the left hip is posterior in the lower limb. If the joints of the lower limb are compensating, there is typically more strain on the right knee and left ankle. In the upper limb, if the right shoulder is anterior, the left carrying angle will be greater, and the right wrist is part of that compensation pattern.

With this basic compensation map, practitioners should be able to palpate any part of the body and hypothesize what is happening throughout the rest of it. Of course, there are different potentials within this model, but it offers a place to start. Even before determining the best course of treatment, practitioners are deciding what and how to treat based on this model. The model can then be divided along its organic and autonomic influences quite easily. With respect to the organ field, we commonly would be able to correlate and identify lesion potentials that correlate with the left lung, the liver on the right, and the sigmoid colon on the left. The torsional strains through these vectors also can be reflected in the autonomic distribution, where heart and lung are affected on the left between D1-4, the liver and GI between D5-9, and the lower GI from D10-L2, and S2-4.

Primary, Secondary, Tertiary Lesions with Compensation and by Level of Tissues in Lesion

If we stay in the somatic field for the sake of convenience, we will see that if a patient presents with a chronic lesion at the left ankle, practitioners would automatically look to see the motion potential at the right knee, the left SI, the TL and the right shoulder, and should expect a global sidebend to the left in the lower cervical complex. As they explore the body in these key transition zones, they should be looking for what moves the least in relation to everything else. It could be that the left ankle, the right knee, and the left hip are most in lesion. Yet if the hip reveals the greatest restriction, then the ankle, and then the knee, the order of priority in treatment, should the lesion pattern allow it, would be to treat the hip first, then the ankle, and then the knee (if necessary).

If the motion testing had revealed a different lesion pattern, then the order of the treatment would reflect that. For instance, if the greatest motion restrictions were found, in order of severity, in the left ankle, the left hip, and the right shoulder, those would be our key areas of sequential interest. Practitioners can learn a great deal about the levels of complexity of their treatments through their patient intake, and note if the lesions presented mirror or reflect, in any way, the pathologies the patient may be suffering. If there is any discrepancy between the physiological expression and the mechanical lesion, practitioners will know, by having a general knowledge of the autonomic distribution, that there could be compensation lesioning within the compensated pattern that is worth exploring.

By going from the mechanical to the physiological, practitioners are never in doubt about what to assess next in their treatment. They are given a blueprint to determine the effective influence of their treatments in other ways, which, again, is reflected in the mechanics. If practitioners are treating *to* the lesion, they may begin at the tertiary and secondary before addressing the primary—a methodology that is particularly useful in acute cases. If the primary lesion has improved at all owing to the correction of the other two lesions, this indicates that the therapeutic effect on the entire body will be greater than the simple application of treatment to two isolated areas. The same is true if practitioners treat *from* the lesion, whereby the primary is treated first, and after doing so they note improvement in the secondary and tertiary lesions. Of course, practitioners do not have to limit their treatment to three areas. They may wish to explore this principle more locally and focally, as they should, depending on the therapy prescribed to the patient. This is where we are able to use our understanding of global, local, and focal.

If practitioners first address the global primary, secondary, and tertiary lesions during their initial treatments, and the body does not fully improve, then a more local intervention may be needed. For example, if the patient was not improving, it might be worth paying more attention to each of the spinal arches in relation to the lesion pattern. Here, as we have suggested, they may look at the top, middle, and bottom of an arch to see what may be influencing any of the three major pivots in the spine (CT, TL, LS). Should any lesioning persist within that local area, practitioners have the option to see if one particular spinal facet is influencing the greater lesion picture.

Assessment of the primary, secondary, and tertiary lesioning is amalgamated into the palpatory exercise of determining what layer of tissue is in lesion with respect to global, local, and focal lesions. If a patient presents with three key lesions, practitioners should be identifying which layer the lesion is on, and which one is creating the greatest level of bind. They should ask: Is it the fascial layer? The muscular? The ligamentous? The articular? In our example above, the right shoulder may be restricted by a long, lateral fascial bind down to the xiphoid process, while the left hip contains a thickening of the ligaments, and the ankle has undergone histological changes to the bone matrix that makes up its joints. In determining the extent of motion restriction to each of these tissues, practitioners are then able to choose the best tool for the job.

3.3 Evolving the Approach

Transparency in Our Approach

It has long been our desire to move away from protocols like general treatments as they are often—due to no fault of their own—misunderstood even by those who study them closely. These types of practices can lead participants down a convoluted path of uncertainty. If we take this path, any meaningful dialogue about the nature of the osteopathic lesion, particularly how it might be addressed according to global, local, and focal treatment approaches, is not possible. We would like to reiterate our purposes in using a general treatment in order to discuss the advantages and disadvantages each position affords practitioners as we move towards the application of collective treatment. As generalists do not regard any one aspect of osteopathy as superior to another, we learn many models from which to distill the principles of treatment so that practitioners may apply what is useful over what is mandated by a routine. In an educational setting, a general treatment can be useful for those junior practitioners developing motor skills that are necessary for improving the quality of assessment and the delivery of treatment. In this way, practitioners can learn how to deliver the correct forces on the correct axes and planes, using long and short levers, in each and every position.

Advantages and Disadvantages of Different Position

Discussing the advantages and disadvantages of positions offers new practitioners a compendium of assessment positions available to them. It also allows them to improvise when they have patients unable to sit or lay down in certain poses. In this section we cover the following positions: *supine*, *prone*, *lateral recumbent*, and *seated*.

First, the *supine position* is ideal for addressing lesions in flexion/extension. It is also ideal in noting peripheral motion restrictions of the limbs in most directions. With respect to the external frame, we are able to note that as we bring the limbs off the table, we are indirectly positioned to the anterior musculature, while also being directly positioned to the posterior musculature. Practitioners are then able to think about lines of force impacting the external frame, and explore the different types of compensation in order to build a lesion picture.

In the supine position, the tension on the peripheral—or lateral lines within the external frame of our polygon model—are being addressed. This helps to take tension off the spine, which, in this position, is abated in most instances by its location on the table. The position also helps for mobilizing diaphragms and moving fluid between horizontal transitions within the body. Finally, we are able to palpate the visceral field; noting any tissue texture changes here can help with our differential diagnosis of the lesion. As practitioners take tension off the axial frame, the picture becomes clearer in different positions (such as prone).

Next is the *prone position* which exposes the motor line, as well as the SI joints and the posterior attachments, to the femoral head. From here, operators can work to coordinate the arches of the spine, including the transition zones that have a significant impact on autonomic expression. They are then able to deduce the nature of the lesion to a greater extent. If there is a lack of coordination of the group curves and the tension from the external frame has been reduced, there could be a mechanical encumbrance creating a fault-line whereby gravity is loading something in the organic field (rather than on the osseous structures). If there is segmental lesioning, perhaps there could be a viscerosomatic or autonomic lesion generating a holding pattern that needs to be addressed.

In *lateral recumbent position*, the operator has many options but finds the greatest efficacy in working through torsions. For our discussion here, however, we will focus on its utility for testing and synchronizing the upper and lower girdles. Globally, the position requires integration whereby the internal and external frames can be coordinated to work together. Locally and focally, the operator is able to address each limb, the high side of the thorax, and the ribs. If the patient is then returned to the supine position, operators can check the motor and visceral response to changes made in all positions (up to this point) via the limbs and viscera. It also enables the operator to address the cervicals and the position of the head.

The *seated position* is one that gives the operator full range of flexion/extension, sidebending/rotation of the spine, and access to the upper limbs. Here the patient's body is loaded under gravity, engaging the proprioceptors to help integrate all of the changes made during the course of treatment. It promotes drainage and helps return homeostatic balance between all the fluid and gaseous systems in the body. It might be difficult for early practitioners to utilize correctly, but for experienced osteopaths this position can be of great benefit to them and their patients.

These positions can be reasoned into different algorithms for general or specific treatment, as practitioners see fit. Practitioners should seek to master each position in order to best diagnose and treat the lesion pattern presented to them. As their ability to read the body osteopathically develops over time, practitioners will accomplish more with less labour, which is critical to having a long and distinguished career.

3.4 Context for Modern Practitioners

Context is paramount when talking about the classical literature of osteopathy. The discussion should focus on principles but many schools of thought fixate on what appeals best to them. We need to know and apply all the approaches that are based on functional anatomy over a long and studious career. Quality operators will have access to all aspects of osteopathy, not just some. It is a mistake to think of doing only cranial, only visceral, or only general treatment. We need to be adaptable in our evolving understanding of the principles. To this effect, we situate ourselves as generalists. We need to be able to treat the body with the best tools available and in any position. This is what the founding osteopaths did over a hundred years ago, and we want the same success for our readers.

As skill level improves, new practitioners will begin to understand how to reproduce the advantages of each position, either based on their approach and/or the limitations of the patient. This is where real osteopathic thinking flourishes, and the possibilities for the expression of treatment become a rich tapestry for exploration. Rather than being a series of orthopaedic manipulations in successive positions, operators are able to address the key and supporting lesion patterns along the appropriate lines of force in all positions. They will look for ascending and descending lesions; they will determine if they are simple or complex chain lesions; they will know, based on their palpation and understanding of mechanics and anatomy, how to treat through principles; and they will trust that the body will do the rest.

It is our hope that categories like general, classical, and eclectic all become outdated remnants of the past and that real osteopathy will endure by its own merit. As fragmented as we have become, we see a way of uniting our cause and returning to our position as legitimate healthcare providers, all without having to compromise our principles, research practices, or results. This next phase of osteopathy will show its maturity as a medical practice and, hopefully, lead to a more united vision of what is globally possible for this science.

3.5 Characteristics of Osteopathic Treatment

Many people talk about osteopathy, but not everyone tries to define the characteristics of osteopathic treatment. This is a mistake because if we think of chiropractic treatment, massage, or physiotherapy, we can conjure an image of what each of these practices entail. Because osteopathy is so all-encompassing, it is more difficult to render a clear image of the practice. Yet that does not mean we should not try to clarify it through the benefits of its application. When we speak of osteopathy in terms of treatment, the picture becomes clearer. Treatment should reduce stimulation and be relaxing; it should be inhibitory to the nervous system and enjoyable. It should not be too protracted—indeed, it should be only as long as it needs to be—and, most importantly, it should have a rhythm to it.

A Mental Rhythm

It is true that treatment can yield results through direct manipulation in an almost orthopaedic way, but that is not all we are after. This is not because we hold a contrary ideological belief, but because of the limited success these types of approaches yield. Treatment without asking the necessary questions and formulating the whole picture of the body does not prioritize the degrees of lesions, and it does not look to integrate and stabilize the changes made. It has no logical sequence, no rhythm of thought that works through the body layer by layer. Without ideas of sequencing, there is no order. Rhythm itself is an ordering principle as it establishes continuity where there is discord. That reconstituting factor should be what defines the characteristics of treatment. For us, based on our proposed methodology, there is a mental rhythm that coalesces through the application of adjustment, one that harmonizes with the quality of that adjustment. Over time, this rhythm is what distinguishes one practitioner from another. It is the meticulous application of a thought process throughout the body, a narrative authored by both practitioner and patient.

Indeed, treatment should have a rhythm; otherwise it has nothing to define it. Without such a characteristic, there are limited opportunities of expression for the operator and there is nothing that makes the treatment their own. More than this, we want our treatment to appeal directly to the higher centres, which greatly influence the health of patients. The application of rhythm in the exchanges and crossovers from one position to the next—indeed, the overall application of treatment—has a cumulative effect that is greater than the sum of its manipulations.

Rhythm is intrinsic to the principles and methodologies we use in our treatments. It is important for integration. It appeals to the limbic system collectively. If it is utilized with the correct application of force—short or long lever—the body will not guard itself and so allow for the adjustment to be made more readily within the mental, autonomic, and endocrine systems. The rhythm, then, becomes an interface that connects the patient to the practitioner, lowering resistance to palpation and yielding a better quality of diagnosis. The patient's body, simply put, is much more responsive to treatment. This does not mean that the rhythm is the same throughout a treatment. The tempo in the application of rhythm can change depending palpation, and that can have everything to do with the type of lesion being presented, the structure and function of the body part being assessed, and the best course of correction as dictated by the lesion.

Rhythm in Handling

Rhythm should also be evident in the practitioner's handing of their patients. Finding the right rhythm is about knowing the pace to use for the patient, the position, the lesion, and the best way to move through the body to affect the systems mentioned above. For instance, when using oscillation with a long lever supine leg rotation, the rhythm is facilitated by the thoracic curve (which is pinned by the table) due to the reversal of the lumbar curve into the thoracic. This creates a fixed point, whereby we are able to assess the lower polygon and gain an understanding—due to its own size, mass, and anatomical structure—of how the structure is functioning in relation to its mechanical parts. We are able to see what segments are or are not opening and closing in the lumbar spine. Likewise, we are also able to asses which SI joint is or is not opening and closing. Ultimately, we get to see how all of these joints are working collectively in synchronization or discord. This makes us more efficient in our application of treatment, for we do not make an adjustment orthopaedically; we make the adjustment because of how we know it will influence all other structures, both mechanically and neuro-physiologically.

Continuing with our example of the leg, as we initially impel the limb through its full range of motion, the degree of tissue texture changes from a lesion has a profound effect on the rhythmic functionality of the hip joint and lower polygon. Practitioners then use their technical skill, knowledge of anatomy, and clinical experience to help synchronize all of the moving parts that are made available by the position of the patient and the application of treatment. It is not just a long lever adjustment to an SI joint or to L5/S1; indeed, the long lever, in this position, articulates and brings together everything from the femoral head to L5/S1 and to D12. Oftentimes, because of the application of rhythm in this approach to treatment, a compensating lesion in the upper girdle will also release as the force acting on the fixed site of interaction between the lumbar and thoracic curves is reduced.

Influence of Mechanics on Rhythm

Each joint has its own rhythm and its own functional complexity that needs to be synchronized. We use the joint's own rhythmic character to perform this task. That rhythmic characteristic—essentially, how the anatomy affords movement—is inherent in the mechanics. Whereas we are able to articulate the lower girdle directly, for example, the application for articulation of the upper girdle is quite different. That variance, of course, depends on the principle of structure/function.

Let us now use the example of a rhythmic approach with the upper girdle in supine position. As the long lever cannot be used to articulate the spine directly, practitioners can work instead from the soft tissues to pull on the hard tissues; this helps to align the upper girdles with one another (which, as we have learned, has an effect on the lower girdles). Rhythm is applied in the application of treatment also, but its usage is from the soft tissue to the hard. Thus, the action of moving the scapulothoracic joint up and down and around the thoracic cage influences the upper T-line with respect to its position of inclination/declination on an A/P axis, its rotation around a vertical axis, and its coordination with the other girdles (whether the lesion pattern be compensating or not).

With this knowledge, we are able to coordinate the left/right and upper/lower girdles because the principle of rhythm application can be linked to natural ambulation cycles of the body during its gait cycle. When there is health, there is mobility without pain. Where there is pain, there is almost always a lack of mobility. That asymmetry in mobility is compromised rhythm, or, to put it in terms we have been using, presents itself as a lack of synchronization between the girdles. A lesion, therefore, is a fixed point within the rhythmic motion of the body. That fixed point—what we call the key lesion—creates pathological axes that radiate altered lines of force from it, irritating other areas, which then become holding patterns of fixations that feed off each other.

In the end, it is not that we are treating the T-lines according to sidebending/rotation, declination/inclination, and anterior/posterior exclusively. These might be appropriate places to start when learning algorithms for assessing the body in early education; however, we are talking about the coordination of rhythm and, more specifically, the quality of the lesion that abates the proper rhythm and co-ordination of the girdles. The presentation of the T-lines are resultants, and so should be used to assess the health and vitality of the patient based on the health, mobility, and motility of the body collectively. The correction of the sum of its parts, of which the T-lines are examples, is what levels these lines or at least returns their proper motion, which allows the body to recover its vitality.

It should be remembered that the use of the long lever of the upper limb is only an example. There are times when this will be the best approach, and times when it will either be used as a secondary tool or not at all. In any case, we want to emphasize that the rhythm and use of the long lever is the same for the short lever, and that the goal of treatment is to unlock the primary lesion and its facilitating pattern with the least amount of imposition.

Stay with the Mechanics

It is one thing to talk about looping the physiology of the lesion to trace it through systems, but what does that mean for assessing and treating the body osteopathically? It means that we go back to our mechanics. We superimpose our knowledge of the key pivots on the body. We note their position and condition in relation to the T-lines and the vertical line. We investigate the lines of force acting on these pivots and eventually build a three-dimensional image of the holding pattern causing an asymmetry and/or malfunction of the body. There is a wealth of information garnered from this approach that will save the practitioner time and aggravation. Rather than following the symptomology, we follow the lesion, and seek to help the body return to a sustainable balance.

3.6 Looping the Lesion

Treating To and Away From the Lesion

It is our position that if we look for patterns of lesioning and question why those patterns of dysfunction exist, then we will have a better understanding of what we need to do in order to correct them. If we are not careful and look for a specific treatment for a specific segment without adjusting the area and its relationship with other areas, we can fall into the trap of trying to do something *to* the body rather than working *with* it. As a consequence of focusing on the part instead of the whole, we lose the mental rhythm we are attempting to establish that makes our work osteopathic.

For instance, if a patient comes to the clinic with L5/S1 pain, there are times when all that needs to be done is a specific treatment to that area; other times, however, we will have to work toward that structure with our collective mechanics. Usually when we palpate L5/S1 areas in lesion, inflammation will not necessarily be found. There frequently appears to be splinting and guarding of the tissue, and the lesion might not let us in to do a simple correction. More than this, however, we must be able to identify what has contributed to this crisis in the body, which means we must consider the lines coming off the different mechanical frames and arches of the body. We need to see the area(s) above or below that might be in greater lesion. Attempting to simply correct the position of L5/S1, then, could be a futile effort without the awareness that this area is a part of our baseline for the lower polygon. This baseline, moreover, has a great amount of influence on the other key pivots and their ability to compensate for the lines of force emanating through the body, particularly at the transitional axes of motion between sagittal and transverse planes. The guarding of the superficial muscles, as well as spasms in the deep intrinsic muscles of the structures in lesion, could be the consequence of forces acting *on* the area or *from* the visceral field, and not the cause of dysfunction. It is our mindset—as much as our skill set—that differentiates an osteopath's approach and results from other forms of manual work.

Diagnosis: Palpation and Mechanics

When we talk about diagnosis we are obviously talking about, in one way or another, palpation and one's ability to pick up on the quality of the tissue. When we palpate, we note any *asymmetries*, motion *restrictions*, tissue *texture* abnormalities, and *sensory* changes (ARTS). This acronym is commonly known in modern osteopathic literature, but it does not incorporate the mechanical element that is so critical to an osteopathic diagnosis. That is why we should also consider the mechanical quality of the lesion, its anatomy, the physiology that is affected by any barrier, and the simple or chain lesion that could result.

Find What We Look For

If there is a short pectoral line on the right, it is probable that there could be a problem with the limb and ribs on that side. If there is a problem with the ribs, the spine will also be in lesion. If the spine is in lesion, there will be a problem with the autonomics. If the autonomics are altered together with the anatomy, the osteopathic lesion/disease process has begun. Now readers might think that we are discussing a heart or lung lesion with this example—and it very well could be—but it could also be a digestive issue that is either manifesting from an upper cervical lesion (if it is a descending lesion) or from the lower lumbars and pelvis (if it is an ascending lesion). If we think back to the holding patterns of different lesions discussed in our mechanics, and then reason through the patient's subjective complaints, it is fairly straightforward to trace a pattern expressing digestive dysfunction or a heart condition. If we are following the collective mechanics and our principles of assessment, however, we will continually look to see what else could be influencing, or affected by, the primary area we are investigating. This approach applies to any area of the body, and should be considered when trying to formulate a thorough osteopathic diagnosis of the total lesion pattern.

Coordination through Sequencing Treatment Approaches

Everything begins with diagnosis, and diagnosis works through the way we sequence our treatment. We will speak more on this assertion later, but for now remember that the only difference between diagnosis and treatment is how far we go into the barrier. We can turn diagnosis into treatment at any time, but we must have a reason for doing so. One way of doing this is to transition from a global, local, and focal perspective, or from superficial to deep. As we move through the tissue, we clear each field of lesioning, layer by layer: first the fascia, then to the muscles, then to the ligaments, and then to the joint surfaces. As we remove each layer of lesioning, we reassess to see if the lesion still persists, and only on confirmation of our palpation and motion testing do we proceed to the next layer. Once we have spiralled down to the key lesion, we are able to spiral out again to coordinate and integrate all levels of tissue from deep to superficial.

Anatomy Dictates the Protocol for Principle-Based Treatment

There are three basic principles that can be applied by practitioners in accordance with the barrier model in a *direct, indirect,* or *balanced* approach with either a *lever,* a *wedge,* and/ or a *screw.* It is important to expand on these basic principles, however, so that practitioners are truly able to read and react to the tissues they are palpating in real time. To achieve this, we can follow either a direct or indirect sequence that allows the practitioner to move through the tissue, layer by layer, as dictated by the area of interest.

A direct sequence could make use of the principles and concepts of myofascial release, post-isometric relaxation, and articulation, allowing the penetration of tissues from superficial to deep. This will allow practitioners to coordinate the changes to the entire joint complex, for example, rather than impose treatment on just the ligaments, fascia, or muscles. In an *indirect sequence,* the practitioner might apply the concepts of ligamentous articular strain and/or facilitated positional release. A *balanced* approach might be a combination of all of these principles, keeping in mind that practitioners are working much less on the barrier, either directly or indirectly. With these principles at our disposal, there is nothing that can stop us from transitioning in and out of direct and indirect sequences so as to work through to the primary lesion to reconstitute proper motion. The sequence used, however, is not chosen arbitrarily, but is determined by what we palpate and the effect we want to have on our discoveries.

Example of a Simple Systems Lesion

We have now discussed a way of working through the body based purely on the mechanics while looking for compensation to determine the primary, secondary, and tertiary lesions potentially at play. To truly bring the osteopathic thought process to light, we will now introduce an example from the organic field that shows how our mechanical model can mitigate an acute pathology. Readers should ponder how they can overlay the collective mechanics onto the following example.

If a patient presents with a bladder infection, it could be a urogenital dysfunction. On investigation, we check L4/5 and note that there are tissue texture changes suggestive of lesioning in the autonomics. If that lesion is cleared, but symptoms persist, we must have somewhere else to go with our thinking. From this point, we follow the plumbing of the body to the kidney. We notice that the psoas is catching and irritating the capsule of the kidney. As we look at the lower polygon, we notice a twist at D11/12. By correcting this and coordinating the hard and soft tissues that are under the influence of the lesion, we have followed an ascending complex system lesion, from the physiological expression to the somatic reflex in the nervous system to the mechanics, and, from the mechanics, we reversed all parameters in the disease process in our application of treatment.

As we look more closely at the mechanics and recall our discussion on the key pivots of the body, we note that the transition zones are important viscerally via the autonomics. We know from previous discussions that movement is greater in these areas, so it is logical to assume there would be autonomic expression reflected in the holding patterns of the muscles in these zones. Here we find reflexive positions between the viscerosomatic/somatovisceral lesion complex. The importance of these areas are further compounded by the fact that there are transverse diaphragms that further affect fluid and air dynamics. If the lesion used in the previous example did not release after treating the psoas, it could have been held by the improper functioning of the diaphragm.

In the end, it is not about uncovering which muscle, ligament, articulation, or cell is in lesion for its own sake. The body moves collectively. The more collective our thinking, then, the better we are able to diagnose and become surgical in our approach to treatment. This is again why we tend to go global, local, and focal in our sequencing of treatments. Even if it did occur to us to look to the top of the lower polygon, it could be obstructed from view by another lesion expressing dysfunction at L5/S1. As a result, attempting to treat this area would do little to reconstitute health in the body.

3.7 Levels of Lesioning: Somatic and Organic

As we have reiterated, if the information is not applicable to the clinician, it is of little use. We will now turn to the six different levels of osteopathic lesioning that will be palpable to practitioners and thereby formulate a framework for establishing a way of thinking through the body. There are six levels of osteopathic lesioning that can be divided into two categories: *somatic* and *organic*. For the sake of delineating the terms: "somatic" (or *soma*) refers largely to musculoskeletal dynamics, and "organic" (or the *organ field*) refers to viscera and the processes of the organs. The mediator between these two categories of lesioning is the nervous system. On the somatic side, we use palpation and motion testing to determine the muscular and fascial lesioning from superficial to deep. Next, we evaluate the quality of the articular surfaces of joints and their ligamentous attachments. Finally, we work our way to the osseous lesion, which penetrates to the bones themselves. Depending on what is palpated, we can say that the patient is either partially, mostly, or fully lesioned on the somatic side. A partially lesioned area would be discovered on the muscular level, while a mostly lesioned area would contain both the muscular and ligamentous levels. A fully somatic lesioned area would include all three: muscular, ligamentous, and osseous.

On the organic side of a lesion, we also have three divisions. The first level regards the quality of the functional glandular substances. The second level pertains to vasomotor control. By this, we mean the nutritional and congestive quality of the lesion. If there is not enough blood passing through the lesion, it is lacking nutrifying tissue; if blood cannot leave the area, it would be a congestive dysfunction. The last level of lesioning on the organic side has to do with the regulators, particularly the neuro-regulators. These we see reflected in the soma, signs, and symptoms of the patient.

We must remember, though, that when discussing these exercises of categorization, we are talking about different expressions of a lesion. Our purpose in treatment is to explicate these expressions and remove the reasons why they are present. Of the determining factors for lesioning of these kinds, we have either direct trauma to the tissue, a gravitational loading issue (which is either putting a strain on the somatic, the visceral, or both sides of a lesion), or a congenital condition that compromises either the nutrifying or congestive side of a lesion. During our evaluation and treatment, we must have in our arsenal a methodology for understanding the nature of the cause of lesioning. Treating the liver directly is unnecessary if there has been a load disturbance that, over time, has put congestive strain on the organ's ability to function to its full capacity. Once such a cause is determined, we must then be able to work from the health of the body to its most painful/lesioned parts to return vitality and the potential for longevity.

The Need for an Approach

The body is self-healing and self-regulating. We work with the body to return health and well-being; we do not impose treatment on the body. Should we employ more aggressive methods, patient outcomes could progress rather poorly. It might be too much at the wrong time, leading to aggravation of the condition and/or an inability to stabilize and take on the treatment. This is also why we do not attempt to treat "conditions." We have no treatment protocol for asthma or cancer. This is the realm of allopathy and so should not concern our osteopathic thinking. This line of thinking, for one, could injure the patient and the profession. Secondly, this line of reasoning ignores the acknowledged principle that each individual is different. The conditions for why and how any one person develops an illness in relation to another is so particular that it is a fool's game to attempt to quantify every variation in existence. That is why we treat the patients we have, not patients that exist according to a statistical law of averages. We need our thinking to be particular and our treatment to be specific to *that patient* on *that day*.

3.8 Applied Principles in Diagnosis and Treatment

What's Best for the Patient?

We have provided many examples regarding the divisions within osteopathy, as well as reasons why we believe it is time for those differences to evaporate. We have discussed how adherents to eclectic methods believe they have the best models for treatment, just like those who promote the Body Adjustment. There are also the visceral osteopaths, the cranio-sacral operators, the somato-emotional factions, and even those who appropriate other *ad hoc* modalities and still call it osteopathy. All of them have an opinion, and many misconstrue their specific practice as being the only one. Our intent in pointing out these parochial approaches to the practice is not to be adversarial. On the contrary, we are advocating inclusivity, a perspective that discards the "one way" thinking that pervades and damages osteopathy. As we have explained, most of these schools of thought do have a place in osteopathy and they should be implemented when appropriate. That is why we position ourselves, in the classical way, as generalists.

The truth is this: all perspectives are tools that have value, and, like any good craftsperson, we should use the correct tool at the correct time to effectively influence the health of the patient. We only get to this point, however, if we recognize that sometimes more than one approach is necessary. This means that we need to be allowed to fail with one approach so that we can learn and apply another. We find that a lot of successful clinicians have honed their skills out of sheer frustration if not desperation. They have learned, practiced, modified, and customized many of these perspectives over years of clinical experience.

General Treatments and Principles Alone are Not Enough

If a patient has an L5/S1 lesion, a general treatment tries to get the lesion to release by treating according to a total body lesion scenario. This approach is good for up-building a patient's constitution, but it fails in efficiency for such lesions. Should practitioners be expected to continue with another fifty treatments until the lesion releases? Or can they use their intelligence to think through the anatomy and its lesion pattern and help the patient in five treatments? We think the answer is obvious; at the end of the day, we must employ what is in the best interest of the patient.

The principles are also ineffectual without the correct context; this is why we incorporate collective mechanics, which is based on the functional anatomy, in an integrative way. In truth, the principles are paramount, but they are nothing without the application of reason. That application of reason is expressed through a methodology, which is what strengthens the principles of drainage before supply, and bottom up/centre out. The methodology we outline here is based on our presentation of mechanics and the functional anatomy behind it. We must make this clear again and again, otherwise we lose the opportunity of seeing osteopathy as a science unto itself. If we do not consider this point carefully, we will either apply the principles irrationally or as add-ons to other disciplines (such as physiotherapy, massage, and yoga). While these disciplines should be respected, their perspectives regarding the principles of osteopathy can convolute both their practices and ours.

We raise this concern because we understand that people are quite interested in learning applied osteopathy as a viable medical option for patients. Part of this intense desire, however, brings with it a phobia of learning technique. The avenues for learning osteopathy have not always been accessible—or reputable—in our country because the principles of technique have often been taught out of context. Now that this situation has changed, we want practitioners to know the difference, as Still himself was adamant that students spend countless hours in clinical practice to perfect their techniques. He did this because he knew the dangers of having the application of understanding become a theoretical abstraction of academic posturing based on interpretations of how this or that technique is applied to the principles. Instead, we must remember that we are employed and invested in a manual science, where the maturation of motor skills requires great personal investment and happens over a long period of time. Together with an applied understanding of the principles and methodologies available in osteopathy, these manual skills will vastly improve the outcome for practitioners.

Applied Principles of Technique

By accepting the need for technical skills, it is easier to discuss the acquisition of technique based on principles. The *modus operandi* of the principled approach is to deliver force to make changes based on the functional anatomy, which then liberates the structures responsible for self-healing and self-regulating. It is foolish to have a chart dictating where to apply this technique on which point of the body. Similarly, we do not have a unit on strain/counter-strain as part of a course on neurological technique. Instead, we discuss how we can effect change to the afferent/efferent output of the nervous system as it can be applied to any part of the body.

Once we understand these applications, we can make more effective changes to all parts of the body, and not just to the neurology. We accomplish this by using short and long levers, direct/indirect/balance approaches, amplitude, rate, rhythm, axes, and planes. The qualities are perfected with our knowledge of the functional anatomy and by observing how the body works as a collective unit of function. As we know, the anatomy mirrors the mechanics, which provides a working context for how to view the body in a variety of ways. This is of greater benefit for those learning the breadth and depth of osteopathy because they will be able to layer their anatomical understanding through their palpation of the lines of force and the structures that influence them collectively. In this way, students learn to apply effective treatments sooner than if they were told to learn the anatomy and the principles separately. Here, we offer a logical approach that explains how things work together.

Position to Correction

We should always strive to control the outcome of a *correction*, our ability to position both ourselves and our patients in the "correct" way. When we position to correction, we are thinking of four important factors that help both operators and patients: footwork, holds, fixed points, and the use of levers. This quadripartite principle helps operators get to and stay on the proper plane of correction dictated by the functional anatomy under scrutiny. When we move from our feet, the upper body, limbs, and hands stay soft. This creates a soft contact with the patient that not only increases palpatory senses, but also helps patients accept the touch, relax their postures, and allow operators to work with greater ease. The opportunity to work with a relaxed patient cannot be overestimated as it helps to both assess the lesion and improve the chances to overcome it.

In short, the better our knowledge of the functional anatomy, the better the outcome. From here, practitioners can begin to think of augmenting the expected function of the myology to their corrective advantage. Depending on the position of a joint and/or the fixed points used with a long and/or short lever, practitioners become efficient in their application of leverage to overcome a lesion. With time and experience, practitioners can then move more effortlessly between different approaches to treatment, such as breath assistance, myofascial release (MFR), post-isometric relaxation (PIR), reciprocal inhibition (RI), and crossed-extensor reflex (CER) as required by the level and nature of the lesion. This is quite different than using a standard routine or employing generic points on an anatomical chart for correction. We advocate using the principles of technique from our holds, allowing application to be global, local, and focal, in any position. It is about seeing the body as a collective, three-dimensional unit of function.

No Excuses

To put all of this into practice takes time. Success over the course of one's career is derived from using the knowledge described above with the maturation of palpatory skills. As these skills develop, the operator will know when, where, and how to apply force. They will also have the knowledge to forecast an expected outcome so that the treatment can be measured. Again, this is not an overnight process; effort, training, discipline, diligence, and patience— supplemented by much more than an academic understanding of the principles—is required.

Treatment is a course of decisions. Practitioners must always be thinking at least three steps ahead based on their differential diagnosis. Mentally, their deductive methods must be able to spiral, in three dimensions, from a global, local, and focal perspective of the body and its lesions. They must also be able to infer from their palpation the nature of the lesion—chronic, acute, or chronic acute—and then choose the correct approach for neutralizing that lesion. And they must do all of this within the context of a methodology that is based on practical application, not theoretical hypostatization, of the principles.

We have observed that those who discuss principles more than they practice them can justify why they were or were not successful in treatment. "The body was not ready to receive treatment," they might argue, when in truth they are saying, "I give up." We do not want that experience for our readers. We want our readers to be persistent and find a way to get the job done. We want our readers to have the technical ability and intelligence to realize that, if they are not getting the last ten percent of a lesion, they should look to the anatomy and realize the problem could be rooted elsewhere.

During the course of students' education we provide different ways of applying this spiralling methodology in order to encourage their individual growth as practitioners. Over time, they formulate their own approaches to the lesion and are able to reinforce their application of the principles in a rational way. We can measure the depth of maturation together with the development of palpatory skills. As students move from the BA to other approaches of treatment, their palpation also becomes more sophisticated, progressing from identifying major landmarks to being able to distinguish the type of lesion being palpated, its pathologies, and its duration in the body. We would like to provide an example of what we call functional palpation as a way of seeing how this growth process takes place.

Functional Palpation

What follows is an example of how we can aggregate all of these elements in a practical setting. This example can be explored in any position, but for the sake of this explanation we will consider the patient in prone position. We need to think about positioning at all times according to mechanical principles, applied anatomy, and palpation. This will enhance control, safety, and efficacy in treatment. No matter the position in which we place the patient, we must think of the functional anatomy. If we lay a patient in prone position (into a sphinx pose), we would expect to see extension, as those segments that did not close—bi- or unilaterally—are the ones in lesion.

Depending on the setup, we might expect to find more of a C-curve in sidelying. Similarly, those segments that did not open, bi- or unilaterally, are the ones in lesion. If we note that one side of the lumbar spine opens and the other does not, we can automatically begin to put the lesion pattern, based on our understanding of collective mechanics, between the upper and lower polygon. We can also begin to look at possible physiological expressions globally, locally, and focally, should we need to.

We run our hands down the spine to find an area of greatest restriction. Once we have located this restriction, we must palpate, layer by layer, from superficial to deep, to observe how the tissues respond to motion testing. As we do so, we consider if the lesion is acute, chronic, or chronic acute. We pay attention to its texture, temperature, dampness or dryness, and mobility. If the superficial tissue is most in lesion (based off our static and dynamic testing), we can then apply myofascial release and see if the tissues yield. If they do not, we can then look to the muscular and ligamentous layers, respectively, again applying MFR and/or PIR, noting any changes in the quality of tissue, and thinking of other lines of force that could be influencing it from above or below.

The entire time, we should be building a palpatory picture of how the body is moving or not moving. We are able to logically test other areas as correlated to the area of correction to see if a collective change is being made. If it is not and we have worked down to the joint, perhaps it is a joint lesion that needs to be corrected. If that is not the case, however, perhaps we need to go up the chain and weigh the thorax against our findings in the lumbar spine (a global understanding of collective mechanics), and then move more locally, again working layer by layer through the tissue until the key lesion is uncovered. Of course, this might not happen all in one treatment, but it offers a schema for evaluating how the patient's vitality and constitution are responding to treatment. It lets us know if we should push further or pull back with the intensity of our treatment.

Three Stages of a Lesion

We can often note the value of a principle by its varied application. The concept of global, local, and focal is one such example. Thus far we have presented numerous ways of using this approach in diagnosis and treatment. We can also use it to assess the duration of a lesion as well. The longer a lesion has been around, the more fibrosity is found in the muscles and soft tissue, altering their function. A lesion that has not been there as long will produce more localized pain and contain more fluid. A more focal lesion will be more acute and affect the neurophysiological reflex. In each of these temporal divisions, the body is attempting to stabilize the affected area. The longer a lesion remains, the more the body will work to implement a histological matrix to stabilize the body.

Three Stages of Treatment

To help explain this histological matrix of stabilization, we have laid out three general stages of treatment and how they assist with moving through the body based on osteopathic reasoning and palpatory skills. Each of these stages are also categorized within respective principles of global, local, and focal. In the first stage, we assess the fascia in relation to lines of force and how they affect the functionality of the body. Here, we look and work for compensation—which means that we do not have a true osteopathic diagnosis as this point. It may take several treatments for the body to yield the true cause of dysfunction.

In the meantime, we clear the fields that are influencing and supporting the distortion of health and allow the body to begin to fix itself with renewed vigour. Next, we look at the four quadrants, and within those quadrants, at either an organ or group of spinal segments that could be impeding the health of the patient. This might mean that we note something to be pursued over a course of treatments. Here is where we begin to see the key lesion and its secondary lesions more clearly. Finally, we turn to the localized treatment that is specific to one or two segments. While we can have success by enacting the first and second stage, without the third, the cause will always remain and the effects will continually manifest in one form or another over time. Sometimes there is a final stage in treatment that manifests *after* the localized treatments; this supplemental treatment verifies that the changes made to the body have an integrative and stabilizing effect.

3.9 Closing Remarks

We understand that the application of technical and tactical principles of classical osteopathic treatment take time. We hope readers come away from this project with enough information and inspiration to continue on their desired paths as manual osteopaths. Ultimately, we hope that we have provided practitioners with a mirror through which to reflect their own practice as generalists. We want practitioners to be honest with themselves, and to be willing and able to pursue that last ten percent of a lesion that will make the difference between health and continued disease. We want to inspire practitioners who are self-correcting, resilient, and reflective so that when they fail, they learn from their mistakes. Any growth process can be uncomfortable and awkward, but if practitioners embrace their growing pains, they will find better ways of forging ahead into these frontiers while benefitting their communities.

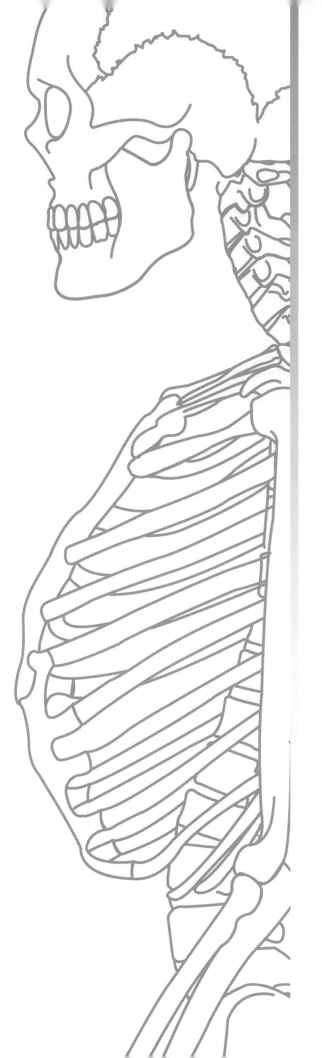

Section IV:

Case Studies

SECTION IV

Case Studies

Now that we have discussed the principles behind some of the basic positions used in treatment, let us now consider some case studies where differential diagnosis is applied. The cases studies are by no means singular guides as *the* way to treat; they are examples of specific patients treated at specific points in time with their own treatment regime. It is our hope that the reader will look beyond the mere description to gauge how the principles of osteopathy are being applied in a thoughtful manner.

Please also note that the case studies are written in a more informal, conversational, *ad hoc* style to simulate (and model) the type of note-taking that might take place when new osteopaths document their own case studies.

Case Study #1

The patient is a female in her early twenties with digestive complaints.

Supine Position

Approaching T-line in this position is all about tractioning the legs. As we traction the leg, we can start to feel where the inclination and declination are situated. In this instance, the patient is anterior on the right. We use this information in tandem with the application of mechanics. Here, we have two horizontal lines (upper and lower T-lines) and a vertical line (down the central axis of the body). This makes it much easier to then correlate the hip with the upper girdle. The anterior right innominate means nothing by itself but by viewing it in relation to something else, we start to get a much clearer picture of what is happening.

As we traction through the legs, there is a drop on the right side, but it feels as though it is coming from sidebend in the lumbars on the right side. We then compare these findings with an assessment of the upper girdles, looking for patterns of compensation. In this particular case, there is a small amount of lesioning on the right girdle but it is not that significant. So although one might say that this could be a non-compensated pattern (we would expect the left girdle to be in lesion if the right hip was in lesion), there is not enough lesioning present to make the case.

The T-line assessment has given a snapshot of what is happening with the patient globally, but we must now look more locally to see how the pelvis, the greatest area of interest thus far, is positioned on a vertical axis. To do this, we note the position of the ASISs, right and left, and see if there is a twist in the pelvis that could be influencing the malposition of the T-lines. There is nothing significant in this case, but the patient is posterior on her left. The next questions we have to ask are: What is holding it there? Is it a mechanical lesion? Is it visceral? These questions give direction as to what to correct first, second, third, and so on. We should customize the treatment in a correlative fashion that is based on the information gathered through the assessment of the patient (rather than performing a sequence of manipulations).

As the visceral field is exposed in this position, the easiest thing to do is to palpate the area more focally and note if there is any tissue texture changes significant to our diagnostic picture. In this particular case, there is a lot of tension along the descending large intestine going down to the sigmoid. The area is also damp and wet. At this point, all indications show there is need for a bowel movement.

Now we need to find out if it is a somatic lesion, visceral lesion, viscerosomatic, ligamentous, or muscular. Remember, we work off a differential diagnosis that is done in a positional sequence, which means that we can attempt to take one possibility out of the equation. The pragmatics of the treatment would dictate that to do this we go straight to the visceral field and see if it makes a change. After taking tension off the colon, the pelvis works better. We gained a positive effect by transitioning something that was restricted in movement to something that is not.

Now, we go through leg rotations. The first turn is diagnosis, and we note there is no lesioning here on the right side, which means we move on. Because we know there is lesioning in the sigmoid colon, we can anticipate lesioning on the left, but there is nothing to be found in this case. Now we know there is a strong visceral component to the lesion because there is nothing in L5/S1, the lumbar plexus, or in the SI and its parasympathetic distributions that are influencing the pelvis. So now we must think about what could be holding this lesion from above. For this, we can defer to our mechanics and note if there is a loading issue resulting from an extension pattern in the spine that is causing the distribution of weight to come down upon the left hip.

Thus far we have shown through our differential diagnosis that the problem with the sigmoid may not be the sigmoid, just as the problem with the intestine may not be a problem with the intestine. It might, in fact, be the thoracic cage, which we can now test. We do not concern ourselves with the feet at this point, as the peripheral joints are about the distribution of force in relation to the vertical line. This is because once we get the centre of gravity where it is supposed to be, the feet will be loaded correctly.

Now we return to the upper T-line and use the first cardinal arm movement to determine the movement of the shoulder girdle around the thorax. We note that the right shoulder and clavicle come off the table. If there is nothing wrong, we move on (we do not go through a routine that "treats" the shoulder). Similar to the lower girdle, we note a minor shoulder restriction as we move away from the table on the left side.

Next, we must figure out the plane of the barrier. To do this, we use the first and second cardinal arm movements. We discover that there is barrier during the P/A motion of the first movement. There are several reasons why this might be the case, one being a concavity on that side of the thoracic wall, which could indicate a concavity in the thoracic spine. We can make this deduction because we know, in this instance, that the scapula must move further from the mid-line every time we bring the arm off the table. Hence, while we are looking at the shoulder girdle, we are also getting a picture as to what the thorax is doing, which will help direct the path of our treatment. We do not spend time on the arm at this point, as we must always go back to our principles and proceed from the centre outwards.

After making sure all the peripheral joints are gapping, we find ourselves at the head of the table where we are able to assess the superior thoracic aperture and cervical spine. Before continuing, it is important to make something clear. We hope the reader sees that we are moving through the body in a way that has a progressive logic to it. Nothing is done arbitrarily or because of rote learning. We do not treat what does not need to be treated; instead, we look for a reason for treating. Given this method, we now come to the top of the table, and we find a glaring lesion on the left OA joint. This has a tremendous effect on the patient's gastro-intestinal tract.

When we began our diagnosis through the limbs, we noted a problem with the GI. As we move through the body, we look for a reason for that GI problem. Now that we are at the OA joint, we apply treatment to see if it will yield; we should then consider what else could be feeding into this lesion between the left SI and the left OA. We begin by thinking about the distribution of the vagus nerve through the cervicals and the upper girdle. We check the upper girdle again, but there is no problem, so it appears that the neck is our major issue. However, we cannot begin treatment just yet.

The neck lesion is a deeper lesion type, but just like with our differential diagnosis of the sigmoid colon, sometimes the neck is not the neck. We must look to what has been driving this lesion because we now know that the lesion pattern is non-compensated between the left hip, the left upper girdle, and the left OA—which is typical of a visceral lesion. At this point we could think that, because the neck is a more significant issue than the shoulder, the neck could be driving the shoulder lesion. Yet that directs our attention to the external frame, and there was no major lesioning in the limbs. Accordingly, our thinking is to remain focused on the internal frame and the motor line of the spine.

Prone

We now need to look at the motor line, so we ask the patient to turn onto her front. We follow principles and go from the base up, noting there is right sidebending in the lumbar spine. Because this is an anterior curve, if we translate it left and right, we will note where it collapses. In this case, it is on the right.

We check the SI joints and femoral heads but, as in supine, there is no major issue here. If there was an issue with the femoral head, there would have also been an issue with gluteus medius and minimus but there is not.

As we motion test through oscillation between the sacrum, lumbars, and thorax, we do note a loss of rhythm, possibly due to the right lumbar sidebending, but we must keep looking to see what could be driving that lesion. To do this, it is important to see how we are testing the lack of synchronicity between the upper and lower polygons. One hand is on the sacrum, which is the bottom primary pivot, while the other hand moves from the middle pivot at D11/12, the meeting point of each polygon, to the CT junction. As we look to these pivots, we think about how each part of each curve—upper, middle, and lower—is responding to its correlate. If we remember the belt analogy we used in our mechanics discussions, we will assess these key areas as they provide a model for seeing how the transition zones between each of the curves is being compromised. Remember: transitions zones are important for several mechanical and physiological reasons.

We need to make sure these transition zones, or the key pivots, are in proper order because they contain diaphragms. Diaphragms have a significant impact on the distribution of fluid, which, in turn, affects the chemical acid balance in the body. This acid balance has a direct impact on the sensory side of the nervous system. So, rather than thinking about having a specific treatment for fluid lesions, we go back to the mechanics, and adjust each of these pivots.

As we look at the lumbar sidebending, we know there is a declination to the T-lines, which, as we discuss in our mechanics, means that the forces that should be emanating through D11/12 have moved (in this case, to the left). Because the pivot is no longer collecting the forces that are supposed to go through it, there is a torsional and gravitational collapse over the gastric field. That torsional strain travels through the mid thorax to get to the lower ribs, which also irritates the autonomic side of the lesion between D5-9.

If we are not careful in palpating the area that is collecting the displaced forces, we may think this is a rib lesion and want to correct it, but now we know that it is simply a resultant of the lesioning in the lumbar curve. If we correct the lumbar curve, the lesion palpated in the thorax will improve. In addition to this, we will also have a positive effect on the SI joints.

When we have a concavity on the right and convexity on the left, we are presented with a question: Is the pelvis right rotated on the thorax, or is the thorax right sidebent on the pelvis? The truth is, it does not matter as the result is the same. What does matter is that we have lumbar sidebending, resulting in a declination on the right shoulder and inclination on the left. This generates a clockwise turn of the upper polygon on top of the lower polygon, causing the translation of force into the rib field. When the turn is clockwise, we end up with lesioning in the liver/gallbladder field; when it is counterclockwise to the left, we have lesioning in the stomach/spleen field.

Remember to look for compensation where we can find it. If there is lumbar sidebending to the right, we would expect to find sidebending to the left somewhere along the thoracic arch. It is very important that we know where to look for this transition, and so, to do this, we look for what is posterior in relation to what is anterior. Going back to the principles laid out in our mechanics chapters, we know that lesioning typically happens either at the top, middle, or bottom on an arch/curve. In this case, we note that the transition happens at the top of the arch (mid-arch) of the thoracic spine. Upon palpation, we find this area to be extremely congested and resistant to movement.

The same principles that applied to looking for global compensation between the two girdles can be applied to group curves and spinal segments. While there are times when we will have overlapping applications, we find clinically that there is much more success in coordinating the upper and lower girdles so that the external forces—due to their muscular attachments that could be acting upon the vertical line (the spine)—are taken out of the equation. If coordination is done early on, a great deal of the compensation patterns within the spinal groupings will clear. This is analogous to taking the wind out of a sail. It might take 2-3 treatments to get the external frame to correct, but we then have a differential diagnosis in play that allows us to see what lesioning in the spine has not been resolved, and we can further address it.

It is important that practitioners ponder this point for a moment. It is natural to want to fix everything all at one time, but we must take the patient's constitution and vitality into consideration. This means we must be careful about the dose and frequency of the treatment. Experience and education give the operator confidence to know that simply recognizing a concavity/convexity relationship, and that thrusting it straight does not equate to treatment. This approach is not sustainable for the patient, particularly if that relationship is stemming from a problem in the shoulder girdle, for example, based on its muscular attachments. Once the external frame has been taken care of and there is no real lesioning in any of the girdles, then we can transition to the posterior motor line (the spine) and correct that. If the treatment does not hold, however, we now know that the problem is more visceral. Had we not engaged this thought process, we never would have been able to isolate and treat the cause of the dysfunction.

As we palpate while using this principle, we should bear in mind the levels of lesioning (as discussed in earlier chapters) from the somatic to the visceral. Remember, the somatic encompasses the superficial tissue, musculature, ligaments and bones—these are all external frame influences on the internal frame. The latter influences our palpation of the skin and the tissues in the somatic field by way of glandular flow, vasomotor, nutritive and congestive lesions, and neuroendocrine regulators.

Supine

In this particular case, we know there is no major lesioning in the limbs. There is some lesioning in the thoracic spine. If we had to prioritize, we would conclude that the OA dysfunction is greater. In our assessment of the arches in prone position, we noted a discord between the transitions of the curves, a lumbar sidebend, and a compensating lesion at the top of the thoracic arch. Very little treatment was given in this position, but when viewing the patient in supine position and checking the OA lesion again, we find quite often that it has diminished.

If the lesion has improved, we must return our attention to the functional anatomy. We know that muscles move in functional groups. As we have taken the tension off the posterior vertical lines through oscillation and/or use of the long lever (whatever is necessary in our findings), the erector spinae mass that acts upon that motor line has less tension, which means there is now less tension on the cervical spine. Now that the external and motor lines have been liberated, we can perform a better adjustment on the neck.

The cervical spine is sidebent, rotated right through the lower complex. We will take care of this before addressing the higher complex and the OA. Here, we begin our treatment. Similar to how we have to prioritize and differentiate between lesions and lesion patterns in our diagnosis, we have to do the same with what and how we treat. We have to know what tool to use—when, why, and in what order. We know for this patient that the neck lesion is the worst lesion.

Our first attempt to treat is conducted through articulation. As we articulate the sidebend, we are also careful to correctly and safely stack the barrier into flexion and extension, depending on how the neck is responding. After treating in this way, we traction back through the neck. Of course we can use the traction for soft tissue, but we are using it here to help integrate the articulation as we are applying this principle to gap the side of the concavity based on our leverage and fixed point.

As we assess the OA lesion, we now note that movement has been restored. There is still the lesion on the left but there is also a large motion restriction as we move into flexion. The reader will note that we are not treating the AA at this time. Time and experience has shown that if the lower complex and the OA joint are adjusted correctly, the AA will typically fall in line; if not, treatment can be applied later.

Once the OA is articulated, we make sure that we also treat the anterior portion of the neck, for it is always important to make sure we treat the entirety of the neck. As we work through our cervical assessment and treatment, we should be mindful not to over-treat the neck. If treated too much, irritation can result. We must also allow the body time to react; the neck needs to respond to the amount of treatment administered to this point.

From here, we could move onto the cranium and note how it might be influencing the neck. In this particular case, however, any lesioning located here is not a major contributor to the condition of the neck.

Lateral Recumbent

From here, we move to the next stage, which is lateral recumbent. We do this for a number of reasons, one of them being the principle that we treat on all planes. The patient is placed, in this instance, on her right side. From here, we motion test to see if the pelvis will sidebend over the lumbar spine, and we note that while the curve will open, it will not close very well. As a result, we will now attempt to sidebend the pelvis over the lumbars in the lateral position, regardless of what we saw in supine. We must treat what we find in the position we find it. At this time, we are not necessarily thinking about using a fixed point here, but about the arch collectively (in essence, inducing a sidebend through its entirety). We check to see if there has been a change.

We now move to the other side, exposing the right lumbar concavity. Although we know we want to correct from the baseline up, we have to consider how that baseline (L5/S1) is being loaded by the spine. We work from a soft tissue perspective, guiding the muscles to pull on the spine and bring out the concavity. By doing this, we are looking to have influence over the coordination of the two polygons at D11/12.

Supine

After making the correction, we return to supine position and we review our work, first by arching through the lower limbs, then by checking the lesion pattern we had found before. For instance, we will want to know if the pattern had any further influence over the cervicals—and it has. There are now better motion dynamics and pliability.

Prone

We transition to the prone position to check whether the confluence of force that had moved into the thorax has returned to where it is supposed to be (at D11/12). Upon palpation, we note there has been dramatic softening along the angle of the ribs, and better rhythm between the lumbar and thoracic spine. As we move to the lumbar spine, we will notice more balance between the soft tissues on the left and the right.

Concluding Notes

It is important to point out that the entire lesion pattern has not necessarily been cleared. We are asserting, however, that the lesion pattern has improved. There has been a palpable change in the quality of the tissue, its rhythm, and coordination. During the time on the table, our job was to remove the lesioning and obstructions that were inhibiting the self-healing and self-regulating mechanisms of the body. With this treatment, we know that these properties have been appropriately stimulated and that the treatment for this patient is about to begin. To perform this type of treatment, practitioners must have an unwavering belief in the body's infinite capacity to heal itself; otherwise, they will be tempted to treat every little lesion that is palpated. In our above example, we did not treat everything but instead prioritized the treatment process through a differential diagnosis, one based on positional and collective assessment and correction of the primary lesion pattern.

Due to the age of the patient, we did not have to administer much treatment, and we would not expect to see this patient too often because her vitality and constitution are still strong. It is a general principle that the older we get, the more treatment we require. That being said, we did not take her vitality as an incentive to hit barriers harder than they needed to be. The application of force was just as much as her body could take—and nothing more. Barriers are in part governed by the art of practice. If this was her first treatment and/or her vitality was not strong, the operator would then apply less treatment and approach the barriers more delicately. Once we see how the body responds, we will be able to give the body what it needs with more precision.

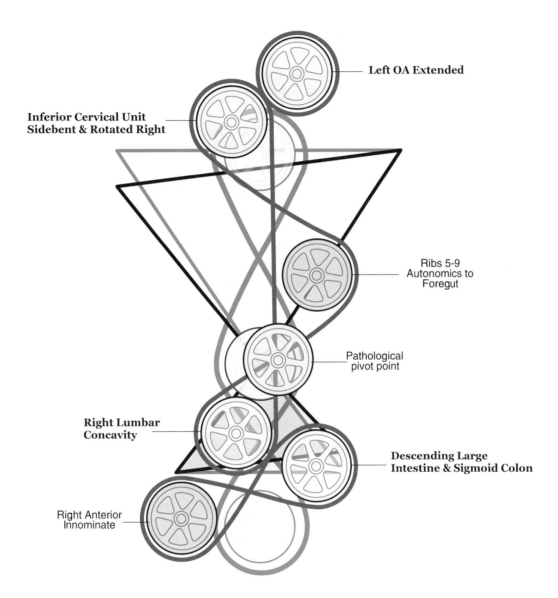

FIG. 38: *Case Study #1.*
• Patient presents with digestive complaints.
• Applying treatment to remove tension upon the descending colon results in more motion through the pelvis.
• Lesion of the left OA affects the vagus nerve and thus has major influence on the GI tract.
• Treatment of the inferior cervical unit (sidebent and rotated right) has a positive effect on motion of the OA joint.
• Lesioning at ribs 5-9 (which is related to the autonomics and to the digestive system). However, with correction of the right lumbar concavity, the rib lesion has softened.

Case Study #2

It is important to remember in osteopathy that we do not always get the patient scenario we want. Lesions do not follow the rules, and as a result, we must continually search for an entry point into treatment. This means that we must be fluid in our approach and make informed decisions based on our findings, the constitution of the patient, and their level of subjective pain. The most important thing for a treatment to be successful is that we make a decision and follow it through. The following is an example of having to switch approaches for a chronic/acute chest pain in the upper thorax.

The patient is guarded. Complexion is sympathetically charged, with mild tremor in arms and legs due to pain. She reports having asthma as a child, and is sensitive to chemicals and smells, especially since having her second child. While the child is healthy, the pregnancy was difficult and the delivery was very quick. Her sleep has been poor since the baby arrived. Deep inhalation is painful.

Supine Position

We stand at the foot of the table and note the breathing pattern and function of the diaphragm; we also see that it is erratic and irregular. There is bloating below the belly button, and we learn through questions that the patient has cold hands and feet, bouts of constipation, low blood pressure, and harsh menstruation. Before moving on, we are thinking of distribution of the vagus nerve, cervical lesioning, as well as any torsion through the lower polygon that could be affecting the quality of blood and its distribution through the portal system. From here, we traction the legs to see if there is a change at the lower T-line, and to get a sense of the neurological tone throughout the body. This gives us our first indicator as a baseline for our differential diagnosis. From here, we need something to compare it to, so we go to the opposite end of the table.

Before reaching the top of the table, we check the pelvis and note a torsion in the baseline that is having an obvious influence on the liver, but here we must be rational and reasonable in our approach. We must make a decision as to whether or not the patient can endure a mechanical-oriented osteopathic treatment, or if they need something specialized to help with their neurological pain. The decision is made to have a more neurophysiological type of treatment, but that does not mean we forget about our mechanical processes, or about our process for establishing a lesion pattern based off a differential diagnosis. It just means the patient might not be in the best position to receive that type of corrective treatment at this particular time. Therefore, we will shorten our leverages.

This is important for dealing with an exceptionally acute patient who is presenting an array of difficulties, such as the inability to breathe without pain. The approach needs to change so that we are able to find a way in. While the lesion pattern is evident enough, choosing to address it directly could have been a mistake, and based on that reasoning, inhibition turned out to be the best way to encourage the somatovisceral reflexes to release. In this way, we are going from the physiological to the mechanical/anatomical, which is the inverse of the preferred method of entering into treatment.

At the head of the table, we attempt to gently arc the upper limbs and note their mobility, as well as the breathing pattern. We check the upper cervical complex and note the splinting of the tissue and apply some inhibition. Through our differential diagnosis, we note that the patient prefers compression to distraction. While doing this, we ask the patient to take slow, gentle breaths, while crossing her arms on her chest, as if to give herself a hug to influence both the vagus and phrenic nerves. As we do this, we note some improvement to the breath cycle. Because the pain in the chest is acute, we next look locally at the upper T-line distally from the shoulders, left and right, to note the glide of the clavicles and their joints. Indirect treatment is given along the left descending line from the neck to the shoulder.

From here, we transition to the cranium to note CSF distribution, as well as flexion/extension lesions that might be compensating for the cervical lesions. At this time, the patient's complexion and upper limbs are flush and the whole body is twitching on the table. To influence the autonomics without touching the neck or the spine, we gently apply inhibition with our thumbs over the eyes, and again, ask the patient to take breath while the spasms are occurring. Once a change in the breath pattern has occurred, we return to the upper cervicals and note if there has been any change to the muscle spinning and the overall tissue texture. The cheeks are still flushed and the sympathetic tone is still high, but the breathing is beginning to improve. At this point, we move to the diaphragm to see if we can have influence there.

Once in this position, we are able to dome the diaphragm to a greater degree, and so we stay in the area and see if we can position the ganglia in and around the cardiac sphincter. We then investigate the liver and the area in which it resides, all the while using respiratory assistance. Here we note further improvement and the patient is beginning to calm. As a result, we move to the top of the table and check to see if the upper T-line has improved by arcing the upper limbs. At this point, we see that the range of motion of the arms has improved.

Prone Position

With the patient more stabilized (but still in pain), we move her to the prone position. From here, we begin by addressing the sacrum, and gain access to the parasympathetic distribution in that area by using overpressure. We note further improvement.

We then move up-table to assess and inhibit the upper dorsals and determine if the tissue is yielding. From here, we position to coordinate the TL and LS junction with overpressure, again using respiratory assistance. After making a change, we move back to the upper dorsals and note that they are in a better condition, and so now inhibit further down the chain.

We return to the sacral area and investigate the pelvic floor to have influence on the ganglion impar. After applying treatment, the patient stops twitching altogether, the skin tone begins to improve, and goose bumps surface on the superior portion of the upper limbs.

Supine Position

After making a change to the overall sympathetic tone of the patient, we return her to the supine position, with knees raised. We move to the top of the table and investigate the oral diaphragm and the trigeminal nerves with overpressure. We then move again to the top of the table to assess the sagittal suture and note the position of the parietal bones. Direct treatment is applied.

Concluding Notes

There are times in practice when a decision has to be made on the type of treatment. This time, the best decision was to perform a neurophysiological style of treatment—but that does not mean we forget our principles or our methodology. In fact, the reader should be able to note from this example that the only difference between this treatment and the former one was that long levers were not involved. The limbs allow access to the autonomic, sympathetic and parasympathetic systems. However, the movement of the limbs would have been too much for this patient to endure at that time. Because she was too acute, a decision to use inhibition and work through the autonomics was used. We knew that we wanted to make a change and what that change would be, and we simply needed to make sure our approach was logical and rational for this particular treatment. In this treatment, we were able to alleviate the patient's acute pain and build an approach that can address the causative factors influencing the neurophysiology of the body.

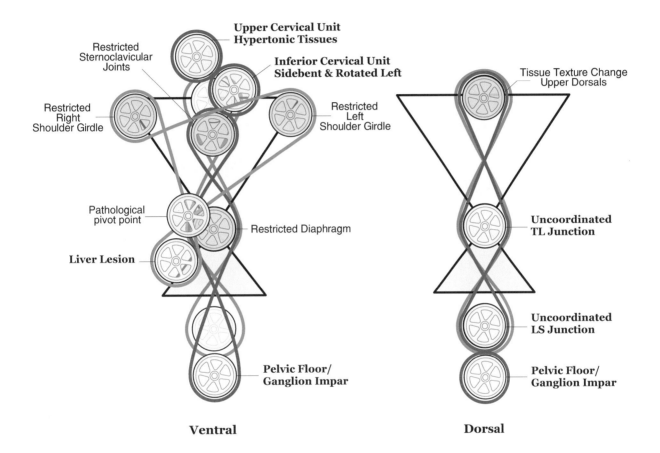

FIG. 39: *Case Study #2.*
• Patient presents as highly sympathetic and acute.
• Through the red belt we see the coordination of the nervous system in order to reduce the patient's sympathetic response. This is achieved mechanically through coordinating junctions, treatment of the pelvic floor, and upper and lower cervical units.
• Through the orange belt we see the connection between the tension around the liver, and the mobility of the shoulder girdles.

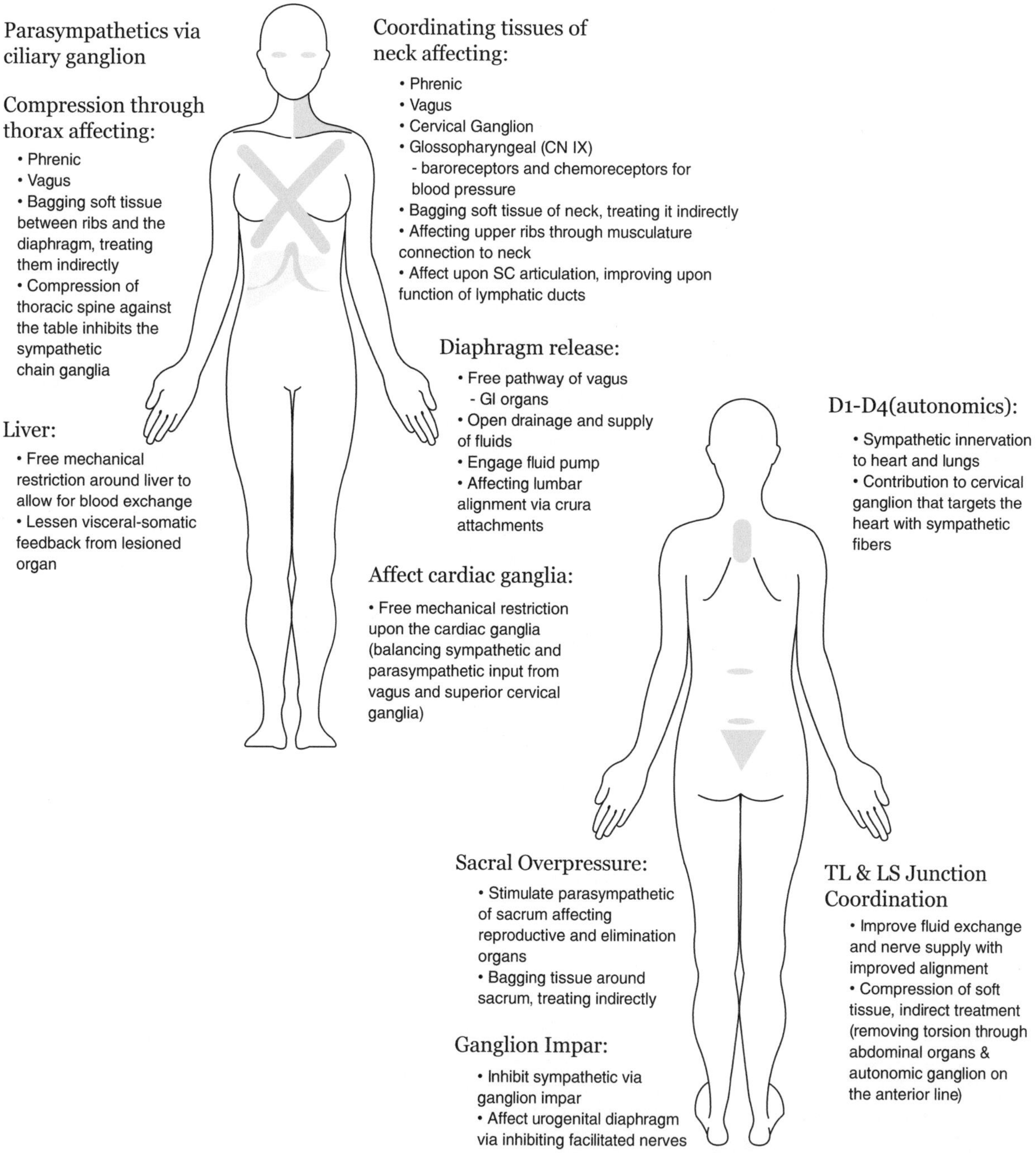

Parasympathetics via ciliary ganglion

Compression through thorax affecting:

- Phrenic
- Vagus
- Bagging soft tissue between ribs and the diaphragm, treating them indirectly
- Compression of thoracic spine against the table inhibits the sympathetic chain ganglia

Liver:

- Free mechanical restriction around liver to allow for blood exchange
- Lessen visceral-somatic feedback from lesioned organ

Coordinating tissues of neck affecting:

- Phrenic
- Vagus
- Cervical Ganglion
- Glossopharyngeal (CN IX)
  - baroreceptors and chemoreceptors for blood pressure
- Bagging soft tissue of neck, treating it indirectly
- Affecting upper ribs through musculature connection to neck
- Affect upon SC articulation, improving upon function of lymphatic ducts

Diaphragm release:

- Free pathway of vagus
  - GI organs
- Open drainage and supply of fluids
- Engage fluid pump
- Affecting lumbar alignment via crura attachments

Affect cardiac ganglia:

- Free mechanical restriction upon the cardiac ganglia (balancing sympathetic and parasympathetic input from vagus and superior cervical ganglia)

D1-D4(autonomics):

- Sympathetic innervation to heart and lungs
- Contribution to cervical ganglion that targets the heart with sympathetic fibers

Sacral Overpressure:

- Stimulate parasympathetic of sacrum affecting reproductive and elimination organs
- Bagging tissue around sacrum, treating indirectly

Ganglion Impar:

- Inhibit sympathetic via ganglion impar
- Affect urogenital diaphragm via inhibiting facilitated nerves

TL & LS Junction Coordination

- Improve fluid exchange and nerve supply with improved alignment
- Compression of soft tissue, indirect treatment (removing torsion through abdominal organs & autonomic ganglion on the anterior line)

FIG. 40: *Case Study #2. Neurophysiological Considerations.* Due to the nature of this case, the neurophysiological treatment considerations should be reflected upon.

Case Study #3

In this example we address the importance of not being too busy in treatment. A "busy" treatment is often indicative of a desperate one. We call it "kitchen sink osteopathy," where practitioners put everything into a treatment, hoping that something will work. Not only is this labour-intensive, but it is less effective for patients and makes it less likely that they will be able to take on the treatment. If we analogize this "kitchen sink" approach to being a mechanic, we do not need to take the engine apart to fix the brakes. We only need to do what it necessary to get the job done. Intelligently thinking our way through a treatment, together with our palpation, tells us *how* to move through the body and *what* work is actually necessary.

The patient is in her mid-twenties and presents with urogenital dysfunction on the vascular side. When we examine her, the most prominent area that is presenting is the lower abdomen and pelvis. There is mechanical lesioning with a twist through the pelvis, extension in the thorax, and an anterior sway of lumbars, compressing the sacrum. This combination often leads to the trapping of blood in the abdomen and heightened sympathetic tone of the vascular beds in the urogenital area.

From this basic pattern, we have enough to begin asking: What is the cause to the lumbar lesion pattern? And on what field did it arise? Is it postural? Is it from the limbs? Is it a GI issue? Is it developmental? While we work through the treatment, we want answers to these types of questions as we assess, treat, and diagnose the primary lesion.

Subjectively, the patient experiences painful menstruation.

Prone Position

We always begin with our T-lines because they lay the foundation for a course of treatment. The pelvis is used as a baseline because of how it affects the central axis and the upper T-line. We start at the pelvis, but that does not mean that direct contact is necessary to affect it. That lower T-line is a diagnostic tool. As we treat the upper T-line, the gastric field, and the limbs, we do so in relation to the influence they may be having on that baseline. Otherwise, we do not have a proper way of assessing and treating, as we have no reasoning to establish our differential diagnosis. Thus, we use our knowledge of anatomy to decipher the functional connections that aid our osteopathic understanding.

For example, with the lumbar extension, we observe a compressive force from the dorsal spine down to the innominates. The effects of this compression will be compounded if there is sidebending/rotation in the compensation pattern of the spine, creating a torsional strain in the position of the pelvis. We can expect this torsion to have a direct impact on the urogenital diaphragm. So we must think of how we are going to get the innominates to move. We know we will have to approach the descending lesion from above, but to do so, we might also have to address the asymmetry in the muscular wall on the pelvic floor, which is attached to the innominates. This muscular attachment also influences the position of the head of the femur. Now, a leg rotation can have much more of a functional influence in its application of treatment should we need it, but this form of reasoning makes the leg rotation that much more effective. It comes down to our intent, which is to play the anatomy off the mechanics to see the body from a three-dimensional perspective. When we are able to do this, we have treatment (otherwise, we have a series of manipulations).

With this type of lesion pattern, we are also thinking of tension in the rhomboids as they gather close to the spine. This means we must also investigate the scapulothoracic joints, which would affect fluid dynamics and combustion, adding to the vascular type of lesioning found in the pelvis. Here, we begin to see the influence of complex chain lesions between the upper and lower polygon. Now, we must find out why: Does it come from the limb? A rib? A lung?

Upon palpation and motion testing, we see that the lumbar spine is posterior left, which lets us know the length and tension on the psoas. This provides a three-dimensional view of the lower polygon, as we are able to see what is happening from the lesser trochanter, around the innominate, and up to D11/12. By addressing these components up to the D11/12 junction, we form an understanding of the baseline in relation to the shoulder line with one movement. We take the twist out of this line from D11/12 down and note a fascial drift on the right. Now we need to know why. Next is an application of our global, local, and focal thinking. We do a global treatment of the pelvis first and see how it reacts. There is some improvement, but we need to build a more comprehensive diagnostic picture. For this, we look to see if the body is compensating.

In most cases, we will have compensation and so we look to the opposite shoulder and see if there is something short on that anterior line. If there is not, we know it is uncompensated and that we have to investigate why that might be the case. Remember, however, that we are investigating in relation to the pelvic sway we have already noted. We do this off the long line (the limbs) and note that there is restriction. After some treatment, we notice a greater deal of unwinding between the upper and lower polygons.

As we reassess the patient, we observe that she positions herself into a lateral C-curve with a lumbar concavity to the left. We push into the concavity to take it out and see how it responds. There is very little movement permitted, so we must continue to work off the external frame in relation to that baseline. We work with this process so that when we get to the sacrum, we know exactly what to do and why. We then want to take out the concavity through the anterior and posterior musculature on the right. After this, we examine the external frame in relation to the baseline—again from the long lateral line from the left shoulder to the hip via latissimus dorsi—and we note lesioning. As we treat this, the C-curve lessens markedly. Now we are ready to begin considering the internal frame and its motor line.

With the myofascial tension off the spine, the spine is prepped for treatment. If we then treat here and everything falls into place, we know the spine was the primary lesion; if treatment has little effect, we know to look further in the visceral field. However, we can only do this through a logical process of elimination.

Lateral Position

From this position, we take a more local approach and take the left rotation out.

Seated Position

We ask the patient to slump into flexion and note what is in extension in a more focal approach. In this case, there is a lesion in and around L2.

Supine Position

In this position, we palpate the visceral field and note lesioning around the liver field. When we ask the patient to arc her arms above her head on the sagittal plane, we see the left is unable to reach the top of the table. We look through the STA and determine there was greater lesioning in the liver field. As we work through the latter, we regain symmetry in the range of motion in the left arm. We then correlate that change with a subsequent assessment of the STA and the symmetry of the upper T-line.

Concluding Notes

Too often, young practitioners want to do too much too quickly. Over time, they learn that there must be logical sequencing, not just within a treatment but over a course of treatment. Everything in this example was well timed and relaxing for the patient. Nothing was forced. The approach is conservative according to some, but not so much as to render no effect. First, the effects of such a treatment are easier to determine; second, there is less discomfort for the patient, which makes the body more receptive to the changes made; and third, the operator is never in the dark about where to go next. The positioning was logical and effective. The patient was not moved into a million different positions. Small pillows were used to help position the patient to correction. The changes that were made were done so in relation to the T-lines. No change was made without referencing these lines.

While there were other treatment options available to us, this one seemed best on this particular day. For instance, the whole treatment could have been done seated, alleviating the longstanding lesions at play through the myofascial structures. We could have used an indirect treatment approach as well, but because of the nature of the lesion, it would have taken longer to resolve the issue. With reference to the barrier, much of the treatment was direct, but we must remember that treating to the bind is a continuum. That is, we treat to the bind in relation to what initiates change in the tissue, and what the patient can endure. With a layered approach and better palpation, we are able to use less force and get better results. Again, it is about being logical and efficient.

Finally, with respect to how to improve one's technical capacity, we recommend keeping a treatment journal. At the end of each treatment, mark down all the things that could have been done more effectively. At the beginning, there might be fifteen different things that could have been done better. Over time, that list gets smaller. At the same time, practitioners become more self-corrective in their approach to treatment, and, as a result, become much more effectual. As they mark down these corrections, operators should not chastise themselves about their imperfections; instead, they should simply go back, make changes, and build confidence over time. Keeping a clinical journal teaches practitioners how to effectively apportion treatment.

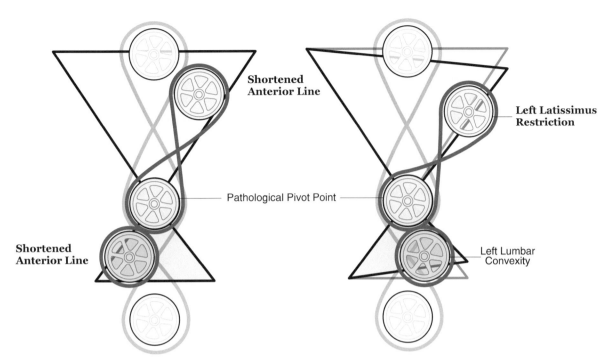

Shortened Anterior Line

Pathological Pivot Point

Shortened Anterior Line

Superficial Lesion Layer

Left Latissimus Restriction

Left Lumbar Convexity

Middle Lesion Layer

FIG. 41: *Case Study #3.*
• Patient presents with a vascular urogenital dysfunction.

Superficial Lesion Layer (upper left): The upper and lower polygons are coordinated by removing the twist at the D/L junction.

Middle Lesion Layer (upper right): Restriction is noted through the lumbar concavity and is improved by working top down and treating the latissimus dorsi.

Deep Lesion Layer (right): Determining the primary lesion as the liver, treatment is applied, which results in an improvement of the STA and left shoulder.

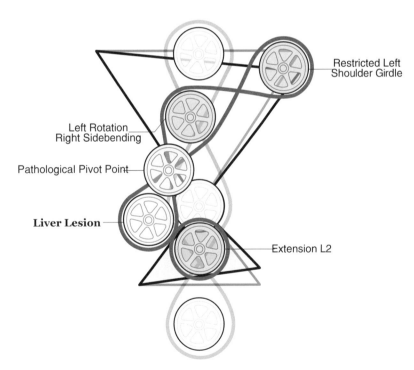

Restricted Left Shoulder Girdle

Left Rotation Right Sidebending

Pathological Pivot Point

Liver Lesion

Extension L2

Deepest Lesion Layer

Case Study #4

As we progress through these case studies, readers have probably noticed that they get shorter and shorter. This is by design, as we want to promote confidence in practitioners' ability to understand and use the concepts and principles of collective mechanics. That means that as we distill the process to its simplest forms, practitioners can reference the contents of the earlier sections to fill in the blanks.

In this case, the patient is suffering from digestive discomfort and is at the midpoint of a treatment cycle.

Supine Position

From the bottom of the table, we look and note if there is a twist in the hips and/or shoulder girdles. We look to see if the patient is breathing well and if the respiratory diaphragm is doming well. We look at the position of the head and neck and identify any asymmetries, and then proceed down the vertical axis. As we go through this process, we are looking to find any major asymmetries that we can then prioritize as primary, secondary, and tertiary.

We note there is restriction of motion in the mid cervicals, and a torsion through the abdominal field in a common compensating pattern. There is external rotation of the right leg and poor motion in both shoulder girdles. As we motion test the hip, we notice bind within the coxofemoral joint. We apply treatment and notice little benefit.

Prone Position

With our differential diagnosis, we turn the patient over into prone position and note the right leg is still in external rotation. In this position, we compare and contrast what we find in supine position to see if the dorsal and ventral sides of the body line up. We spring the spine, comparing left and right, looking for asymmetry and motion restrictions. The greatest motion restriction was in the sacrum. We apply treatment, and check up and down the chain, from the lower limbs all the way along the spine. We go back to our primary lesion in the sacrum and note that it is much better.

Supine Position

Motion restrictions in the upper girdles have much improved and the torsion through the abdominal field has lessened. The greatest motion restriction is now found in the mid cervical spine. We apply treatment and the lumbar spine releases; physiological activity can be observed in the epigastric fossa region, and the patient's breathing becomes much slower and deeper. We check the diaphragm and note that it is moving more symmetrically and with greater ease.

Concluding Notes

This is an example of a rather short treatment relative to the other ones provided, but that does not mean it was any less effective. We must remember this was part of a series of treatments to help the patient regain health.

When the patient first arrived, there was rapid weight loss, poor coordination and ambulation of movement, and dizziness. This patient was treated frequently with an emphasis on the cervical spine and transition zones all the way through the body. When we arrived at this point of her treatment protocol, we noted that there was a longstanding sacral treatment that was most likely driving a great deal of the dysfunction noted upon her arrival to the clinic.

We remember that the lumbar and cervical spine mirror one another; thus, as the cervical lesioning dissipated, the lumbar lesioning also dissipated, that is, until the sacrum was revealed as the anchor to the spine. In this way, the occiput and the sacrum were mirrored as well. Over the course of treatment, the time duration went from 20 minutes to 10 minutes.

The key point for readers to appreciate is that we were able to make many changes by focusing on the structural frame. Through our assessment and treatment we could see a distortion from the keystone in the pelvis. From this boney structure, we were able to influence all the other structures in and around it that work with, and have influence on, other structures in the body.

For example, with our adjustment to the lower polygon, we were able to take tension off the pelvic floor, which functions as a horizontal diaphragm that must work in conjunction with all the other diaphragms in the body. During our treatment and evaluation, we were able to note positive changes in the function of the respiratory diaphragm. We did not apply direct treatment to this area, but, by affecting the boney structure of the lower polygon, we were able to influence the position of the lumbar spine and its attachments. (With respect to the diaphragm, these attachments are shared with the lower ribs.) As a result, we did not need a visceral treatment to treat the viscera; we needed only return to our functional anatomy.

As we received a positive response from the dosage of treatment administered, we did not have to cover every possible position. We know from our principles that a correction in one plane of motion is a correction in all. At the same time, if we did not feel the lesion release, we may have had to test a different position. Yet because we should focus on only doing that which is necessary, we let the body do the rest.

While the right leg was still externally rotated at the end of the treatment, upon testing, we note there is better movement. Improved movement is what we are after, as we do not yet know how longstanding the lesion pattern may be. Because we know the influence of the lumbars and lower limb on the pelvis, we might explore, in subsequent treatments, the potential for descending and/or ascending chain lesions that could be influencing how the sacrum is loading.

Some might argue that we needed to address drainage to the pelvis before making a change. However, there was not a great deal of bogginess in our palpation, and even if there was quite a bit of fluid, our job remains the same. If we do not remove the cause for fluid accumulation in the first place, accumulation will reoccur.

This study provides a fitting example of discipline in treatment. Many practitioners find themselves doing too much for any number of reasons. Some forget that they are providing osteopathic treatment, not selling minutes. Others lack confidence. Furthermore, some are still developing their palpation and, unsure if they have really made a change, keep working away without purpose or direction. Hopefully readers will garner the knowledge, confidence, and experience to know what type of practitioner they want to be.

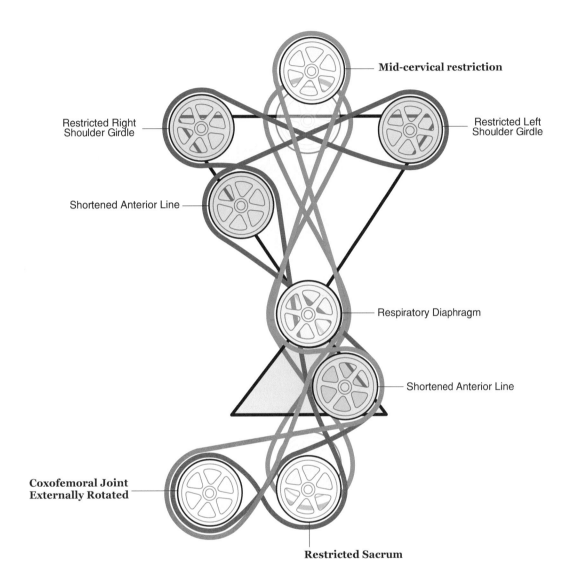

FIG. 42: *Case Study #4.*
• Patient presents with digestive issues.
• The red lesion belt demonstrates the resulting improvement found with correction of the sacral lesion, including improved should girdle motion and lessening of torsion through the abdominal field.
• The orange belt demonstrates the release of the lumbar spine and physiological changes at the epigastric fossa and respiratory diaphragm with correction of the cervical lesion.

Case Study #5

This final case study is actually an algorithm for practitioners to use. It is a chance to practice and formulate how to use a differential diagnosis based on the principles of collective mechanics in assessment and treatment. Over time, their ability to use this information and to prioritize the primary, secondary, and tertiary lesions will improve. So will their ability to spiral from a global, local, and focal perspective, which will aid in deploying the tools for applying treatment.

When using this methodology, it is important to track changes as we go through the body. There is no sense making a change and then not checking our work. As we have iterated again and again, we do not want practitioners to do more than is necessary to yield an effective result. Also, assessments should be consistent with the positions patients are treated in. If assessing and treating the lumbar spine in lateral recumbent, check the area again before moving the patient. It is also a good idea, after practitioners have established their primary, secondary, and tertiary lesions in their initial assessments, to periodically return patients back to that original position to see how the lesions are (or are not) clearing. By doing this, practitioners will become more efficient over time by learning what *did* and *did not* work through the course of their treatments.

As we provide an algorithm for going through the body, readers should remember that what follows is only one possible formula. Practitioners, we hope, will devise their own methodologies and share them with their osteopathic communities.

Proposed Algorithm

1. **What stands out the most?**
   a. Where is the largest asymmetry? The second largest? The third?
   b. Which one moves the least?

2. **Can the patient move, actively and passively?**

3. **What is the mechanical picture of the lesion pattern?**
   a. How does it fit into polygon mechanics (for example)?
   b. Do you see compensation where you should?
   c. Are there ascending and/or descending tracks?
   d. How does the lesion picture correlate between the anatomical, mechanical, physiological and pathophysiological findings?

4. **What is/are the layer(s) of the lesion?**
   a. Is it fascial, muscular, ligamentous, or boney?
   b. What is the best approach to take in treatment?

5. **Apply the treatment dictated by the level of lesioning palpated.**

6. **Does tissue respond? Is there a change?**

7. **How does treatment affect primary lesions? Compensation pattern(s)?**

8. **Repeat the process.**

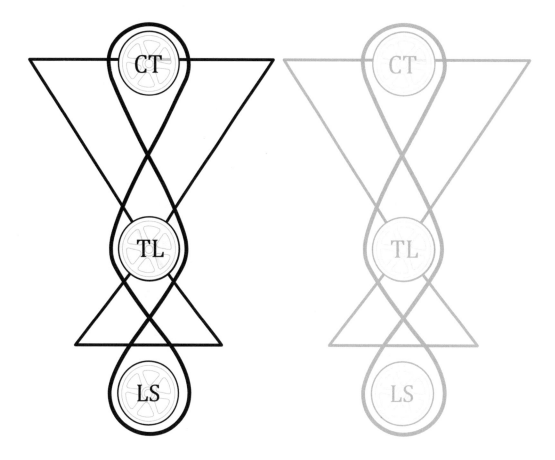

FIG. 43: *Case Study #5.*
These diagrams have been provided for the practitioner's use when applying the treatment algorithm described.

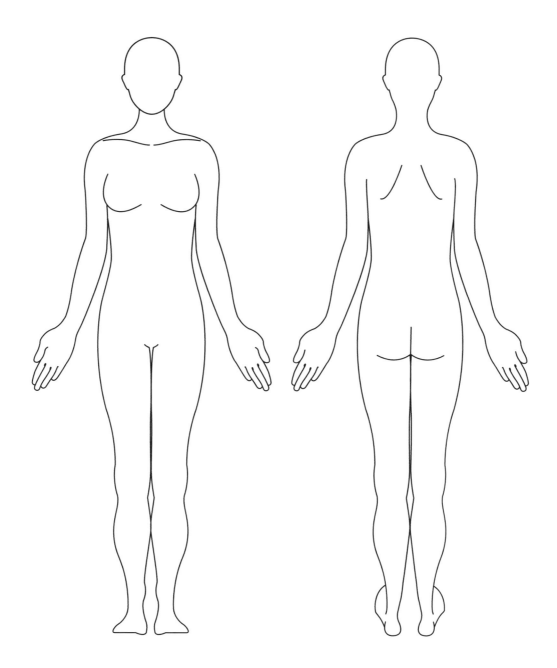

FIG. 43b

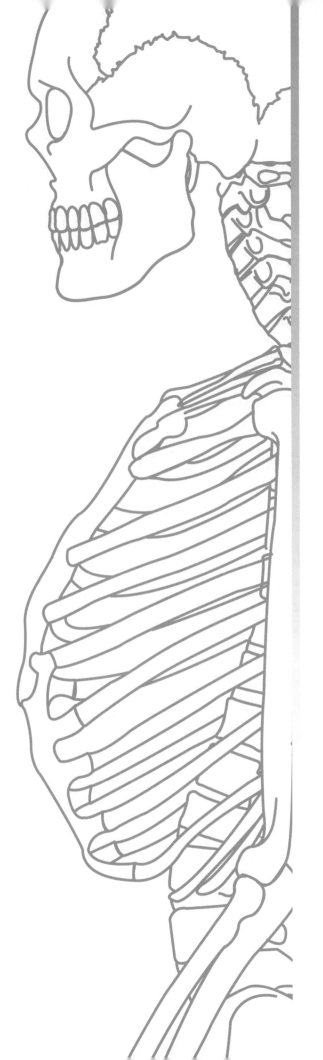

Appendix:

Illustrations

_____ Appendix _____

2.3 The T-Lines

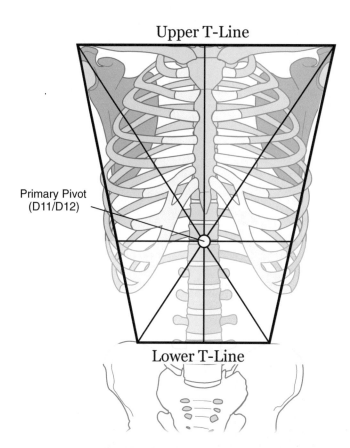

FIG. 1: Here we see the axial skeleton divided into four quadrants on the coronal plane. The T-lines form the top and bottom horizontal lines, and the centre horizontal line is at the level of the primary pivot (D11/12) dorsally, and the epigastric fossa ventrally.

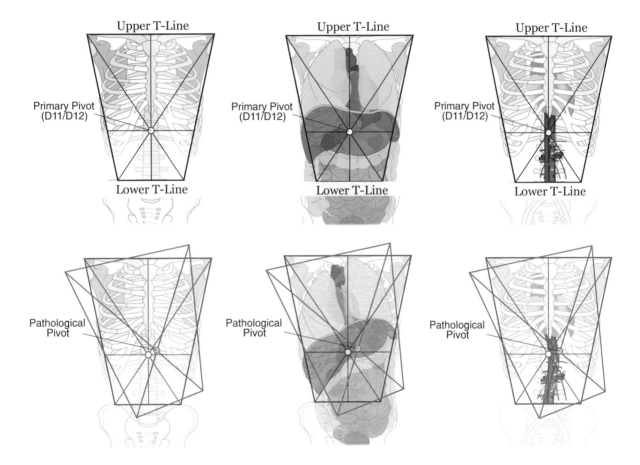

FIG. 2: Here we see the affect caused by asymmetry through the quadrants, and discoordination between the upper and lower girdles throughout the primary pivot. With the primary pivot off of its proper axis, a new mechanical pathological pivot is placed onto other structures, such as a rib head (*left*). In the visceral field, the pathological pivot point can create lesioning within the liver/gallbladder field or the stomach/spleen field. The abnormal forces encourage congestion throughout the organ field, for example, when the right lung compresses the liver (*centre*). The translation of force across the abdominal aorta not only affects the fluid dynamics of the system, but also the prevertebral plexuses of the autonomic nervous system. Tension from the pathological pivot point shown above (*right*) may create abnormal function of the celiac and superior mesenteric plexuses in particular, affecting digestion and elimination functions.

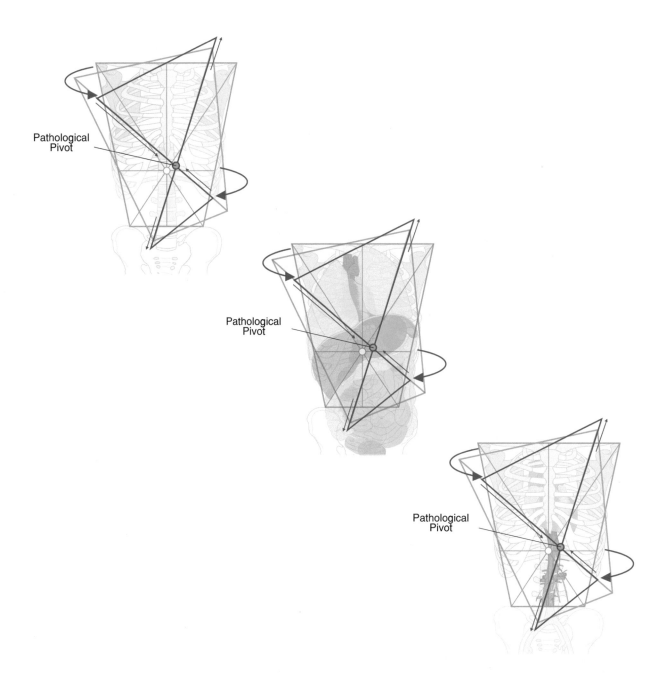

Pathological Pivot

Pathological Pivot

Pathological Pivot

FIG. 3: Here a torsional influence brought about by a typical spinal coupling in the dorsal and lumbar spine has been added. The tension and compressive forces acting upon the organs is further complicated by the added strain coming from the outside, through the limbs.

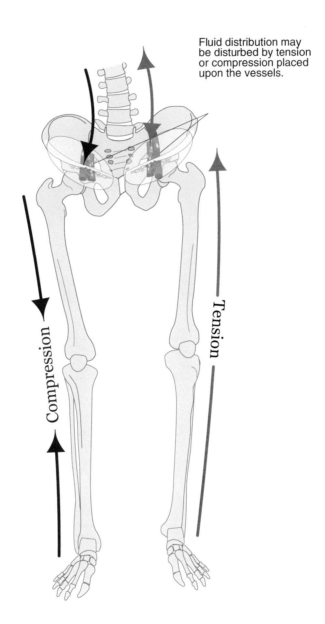

Fluid distribution may
be disturbed by tension
or compression placed
upon the vessels.

Compression

Tension

FIG 4: With an asymmetrical shift at the primary pivot, a limb will express tension and the other compression. This mechanical lesion may lead to a difference in vascular distribution between one leg and the other.

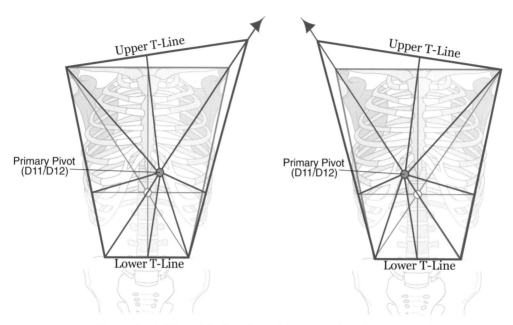

Forces directed through the long lever of the arm to affect the upper quadrants.

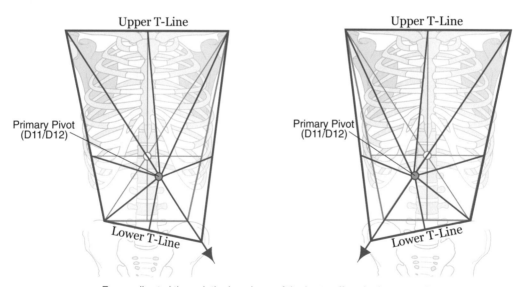

Forces directed through the long lever of the leg to affect the lower quadrants.

FIG. 5: Using functional anatomical connections between each of the four limbs and their corresponding quadrant will affect the alignment of the upper and lower girdles, as well as the primary pivot, through forces applied using the limb as a long lever.

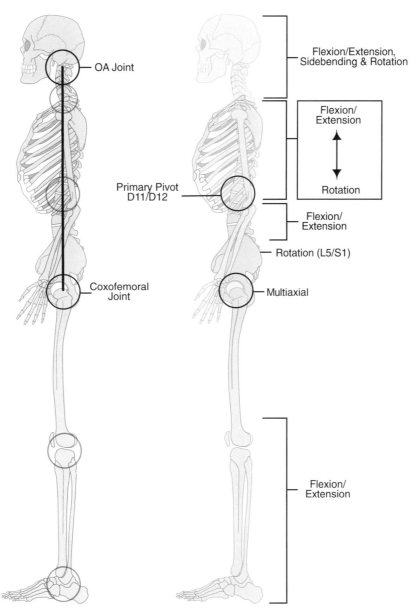

FIG. 6: Two central pivots that should be lined up with one another from the sagittal view—the upper cervical complex, and the coxofemoral joints.

Primary motion:
- Ankle/Knee - Flexion/Extension
- Coxofemoral - Multiaxial
- L5/S1 - Rotation
- Lumbar Spine - Flexion/Extension
- D11/D12 (Primary Pivot) - Rotation
- Lower Thoracic Spine - Rotation
- Upper Thoracic Spine - Flexion/Extension
- Cervical Spine - Flexion/Extension/Sidebending/Rotation

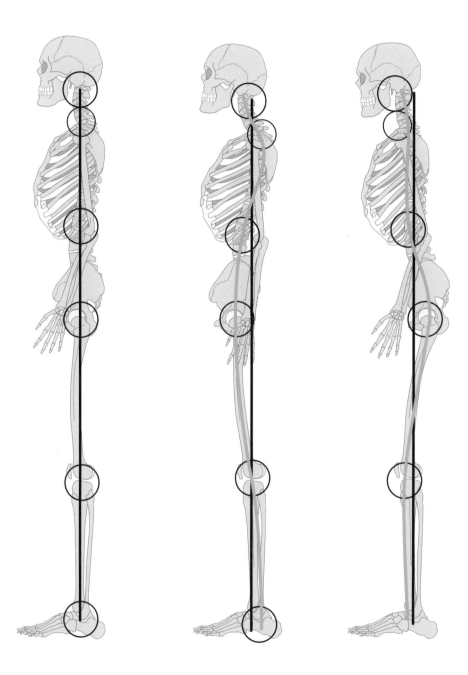

FIG. 7: A comparative illustration between neutral (*left*) and the changed transition of forces through the body in the sagittal plane caused by altered position of the baseline. With the coxofemoral joints translated anteriorly (*centre*), the scapulothoracic joint will pull the thorax back. With the coxofemoral joints translated posteriorly (*right*), the scapulothoracic joint internally rotates using the upper limbs as counterweights.

2.4 From Quadrants to Polygons

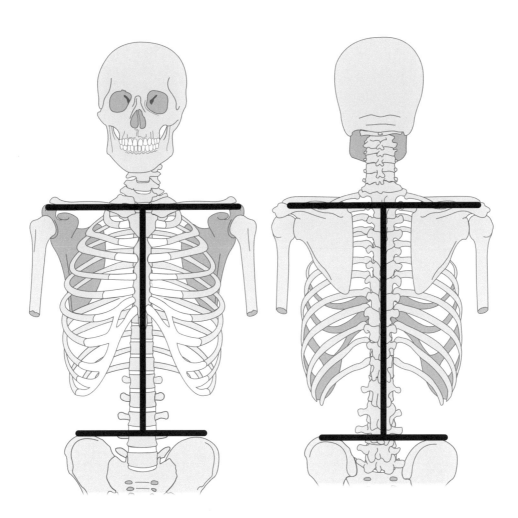

FIG 8: *Hard lines.* Consisting of the central motor line (spine) and the upper and lower T-lines.

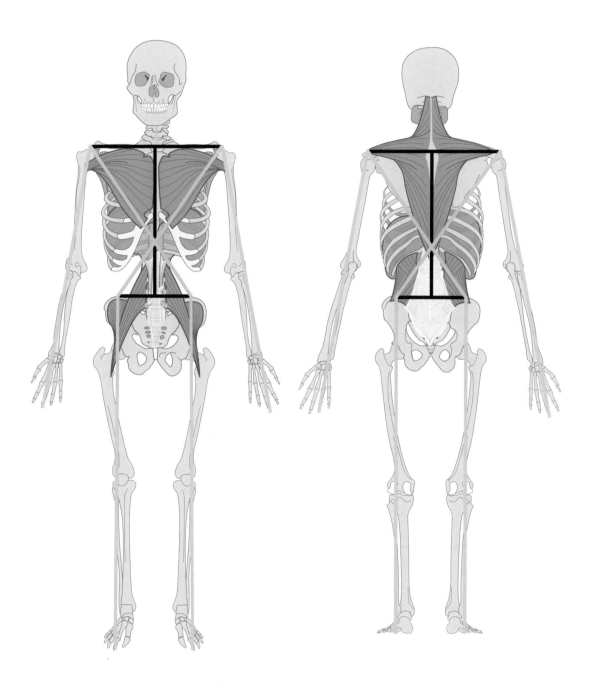

FIG. 9: Here the major muscles that come from the limbs and T-lines and intersect at D11/12 are added on top of the hard lines. Muscles of interest include psoas and pectoralis major on the ventral side, and trapezius and quadratus lumborum on the dorsal side.

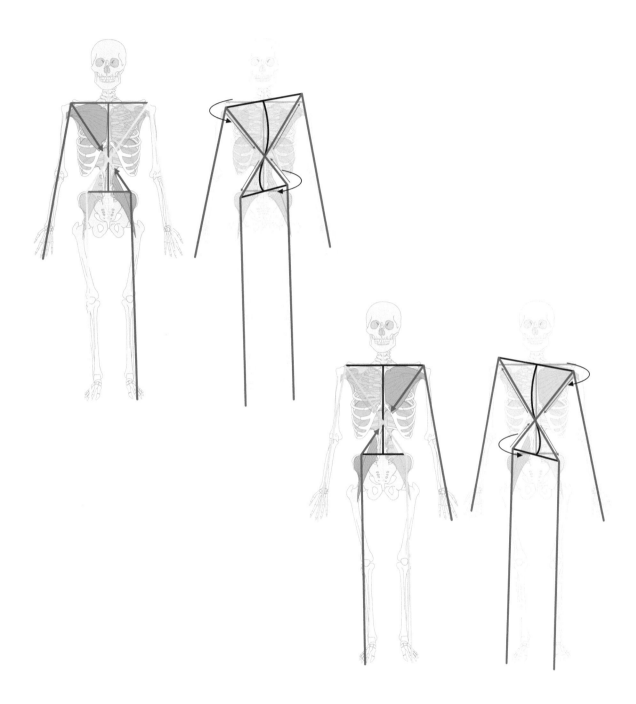

FIG. 10: Here, torsional strains from the upper polygon to the lower polygon are shown on the ventral lines between the psoas muscles and the contralateral pectoralis major.

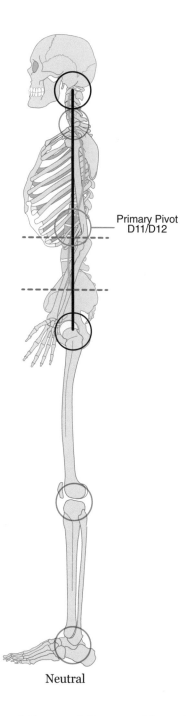

Neutral

FIG. 11: Here we can see the body in a relative neutral alignment, with a vertical line from the upper cervical complex to the coxofemoral joints. Two horizontal divisions isolate the lumbar spine. Within this division are the primary joints for flexion/extension. Sidebending/rotation comes to a point at the primary pivot.

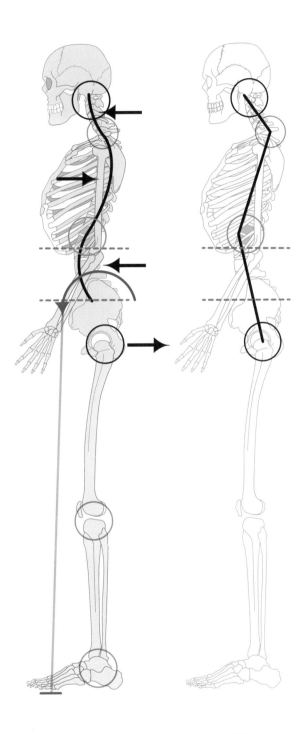

FIG. 12: With a bilateral posterior shift in the CF joints, the lumbars will drift into extension, dropping the dorsal spine into flexion.

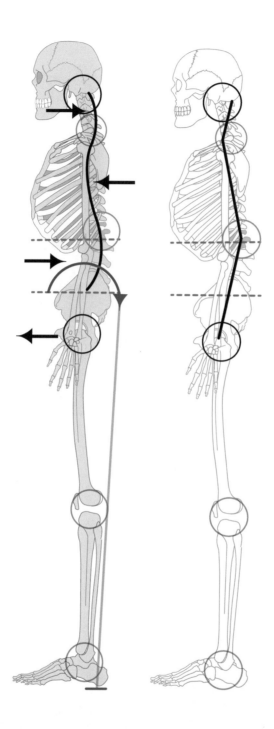

FIG. 13: Here the CF joints are positioned anterior bilaterally, which adjusts the lumbar spine into a flexed position, putting the dorsal spine into extension.

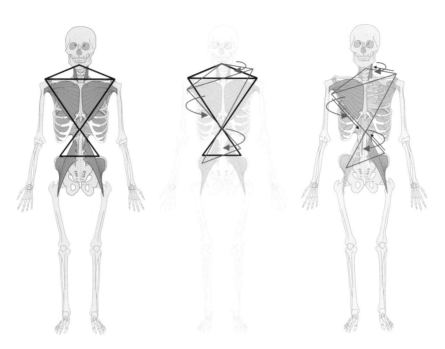

FIG. 14: The unilateral hinge on the soft tissue forms a continuous strain through large muscles that work oblique axes, including the psoas in the lower polygon, the trapezius in the upper polygon, and the trapezius from the upper T-line spanning towards the occiput (*centre*). The sternocleidomastoid mirrors the psoas, going from posterior to anterior, to continue to compensate for the unilateral hinge at the seat of stability (*right*).

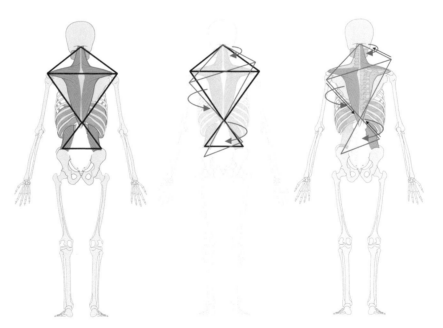

FIG. 14b: The unilateral hinge, dorsal view.

2.5 Polygons to Internal/External Frames and Key Lesions

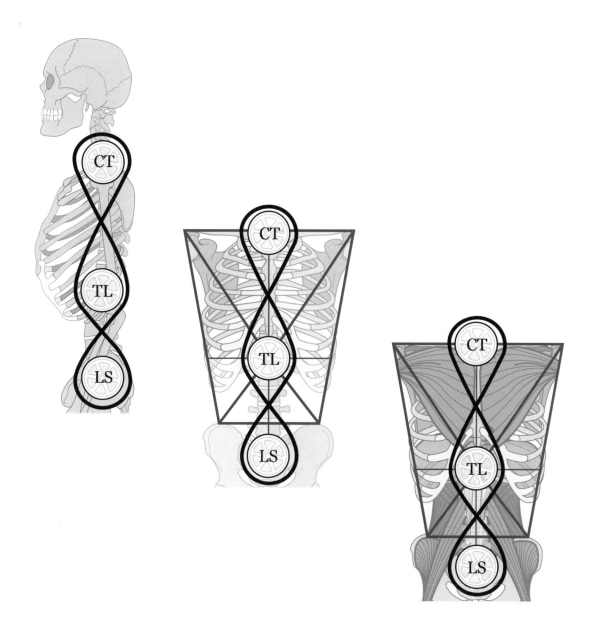

FIG. 15: The four quadrants and the two polygons (upper and lower) are shown in relation to the three key pivots at the cervicothoraco (CT) junction, the thoracolumbar (TL) junction, and the lumbosacral (LS) junction.

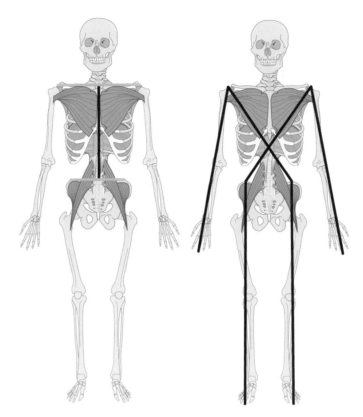

FIG. 16: The lateral lines from the upper and lower T-lines form the External Frame, and the motor line/spinal organ consists of the Internal Frame (*left*). The External Frame follows the limbs into the axial frame to D11/12 (*right*).

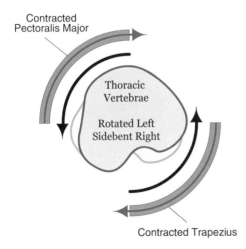

Contracted
Pectoralis Major

Thoracic
Vertebrae

Rotated Left
Sidebent Right

Contracted Trapezius

FIG. 17: The operator may globally address the External Frame in order to better determine the degrees of lesioning in the Internal Frame.

The operator should note that the External Frame may be compensating for the lesion pattern of the Internal Frame. In this case, the operator applies the principle of treating superficial to deep, addressing the soft tissue lines of the External Frame in order to see the deeper lesioning of the osseous Internal Frame.

The illustrated example above shows a left rotation throughout the thoracic vertebrae (osseous to Internal Frame). The soft tissue in the thorax from the External Frame compensates with a right torsion.

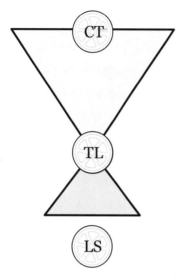

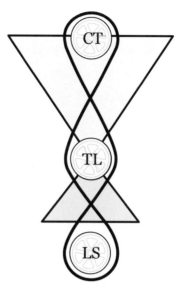

FIG. 18: The CT, TL and LS junctions are pulleys that are unified by the Internal Frame.

FIG. 19: *Belt Loop.* A belt loop around the pulleys shows the dynamic relationship between the Internal and External Frames. When the body is balanced, the tension on the belt is uniform and there is symmetry in position and motion of the upper and lower T-lines and the vertical line.

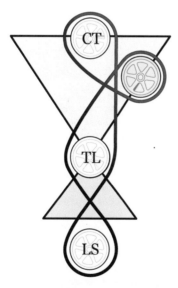

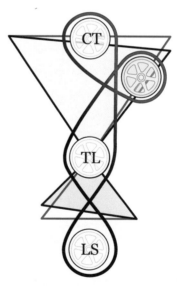

FIG. 20: *Key Lesion.* A key lesion is added to the rib field causing a fixation point. The fixation point becomes a pathological pivot that augments the tension and position of the central belt.

FIG. 21: *Effect on T-Lines & Polygons.* The belt remains the same length; thus the new fixation point causes the belt to pull the T-lines and polygons off their axes. This causes the internal and external frame to become uncoordinated.

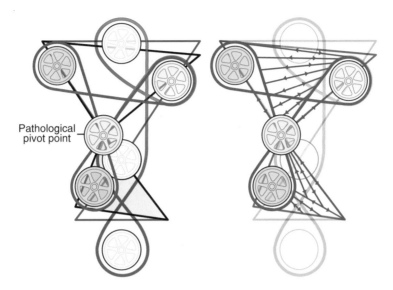

FIG. 22: *Holding Pattern.* The key lesion creates a holding pattern of secondary lesions that facilitate its position. Primary fixations and the facilitating patterns reinforce one another, and the pathological belt system created competes with the physiological belt system.

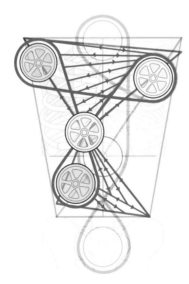

FIG. 23: *Lines of Force.* Lines of force radiate to and from the lesion. We must attempt to return functional symmetry to each of the four quadrants.

2.6 The Spinal Organ and the Buckled Arch

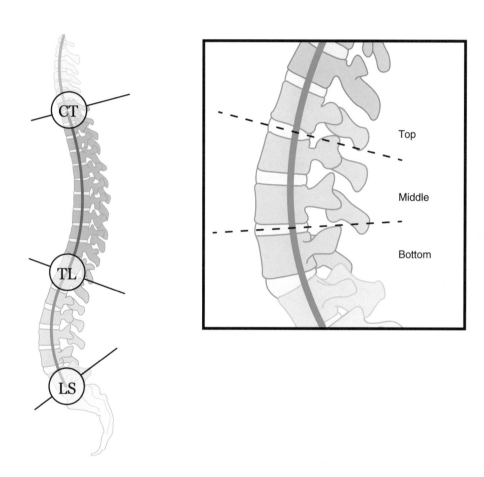

FIG. 24: Each curve, or arch, can be divided into three major sections: the top, middle, and bottom.

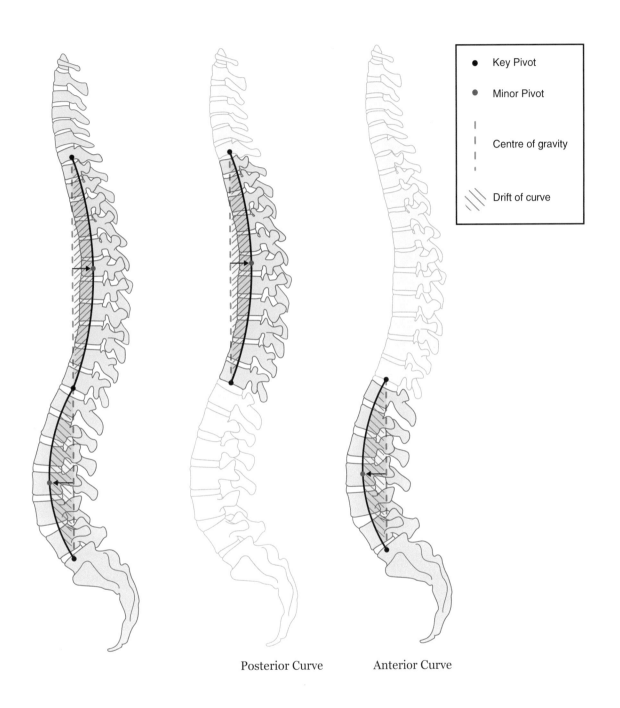

Posterior Curve   Anterior Curve

FIG. 25: *Anterior and posterior curves.*

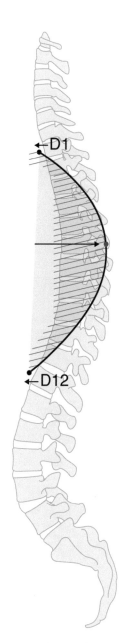

●	Key Pivot
●	Minor Pivot
⬚	Drift of curve

Extension Lesion at D1 and D12

FIG. 26: *Flexion lesion at D6 driven by extension lesions at D1 and D12.*

2.7 The Limbs and Ascending/Descending Lesions

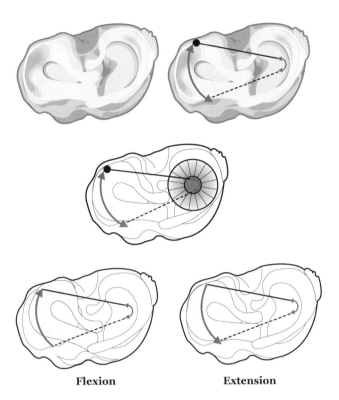

Flexion   **Extension**

In closed chain movement, the motion of the medial condyle of the femur is restricted by the thick medial collateral ligament, creating a pivot point upon the medial tibial plateau.

As the knee flexes and extends, the lateral condyle of the femur and the lateral meniscus shifts posterior and anterior upon the tibial plateau respectively.

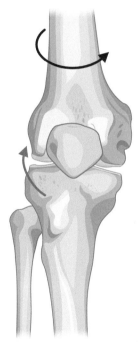

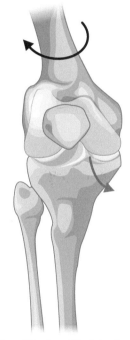

Knee Extension: The lateral condyle of the femur reaches the physiological barrier while the medial condyle of the femur continues moving through its range of motion, creating posterolateral glide of the tibial plateau.

Knee Flexion: The lateral condyle of the femur reaches the physiological barrier while the medial condyle of the femur continues moving through its range of motion, creating anteromedial glide of the tibial plateau.

FIG. 27: The practitioner should look to the why and how of structures in terms of their construction. They should ask, "Why is it structured this way" and "What is that structure best at doing? And why is this so?"

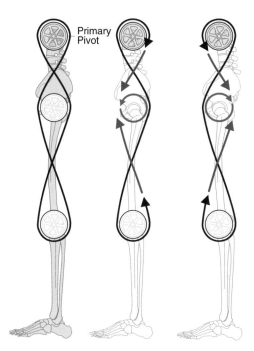

Primary Pivot

FIG. 28: If there is a shift in rotation of the innominate— either flexed or extended—the changes in the tension lines will then cause lesioning in the functioning of the lower limb, such as the knee.

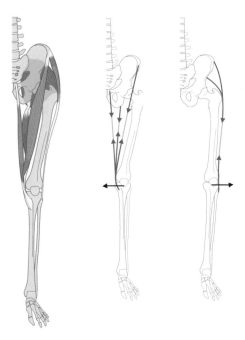

FIG. 29: This diagram shows how the altered axis (resulting from an innominate in the wrong position) will either cause a bilateral or unilateral shear (anterior or posterior) or torsion (internal or external) of the tibial plateau.

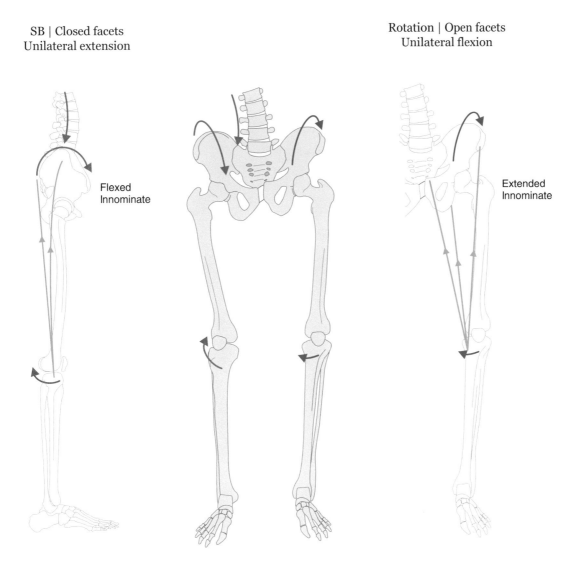

SB | Closed facets
Unilateral extension

Rotation | Open facets
Unilateral flexion

Flexed
Innominate

Extended
Innominate

FIG. 30: The malposition of the innominate can be greatly influenced from above by the lumbar spine. If the lumbars are loaded incorrectly, bi- or unilaterally, we can get bi- or unilateral pelvic tilt. Here we find the lumbar spine sidebending to the right and rotating towards the left. The right innominate will be anterior, and the left, posterior, affecting the tension lines that go down to create a tibial torsion at the knee.

2.8 The Thorax

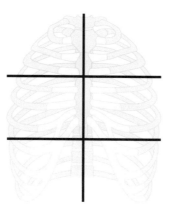

FIG. 31: The thorax divided into six section: the upper ribs, middle and lower ribs on the right and left sides of the thorax.

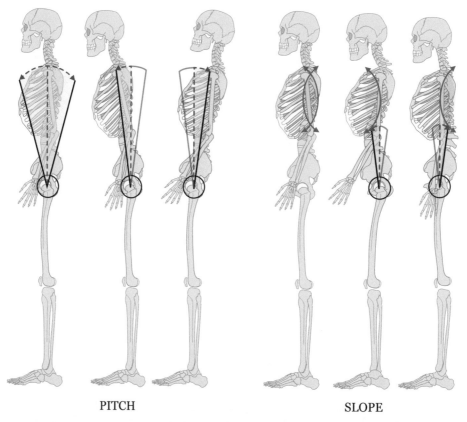

PITCH   SLOPE

FIG. 32: The direction of the slope of the thorax has to do with sidebending and rotation. The pitch, or angulation, of the thorax corresponds to flexion/extension of the pelvis.

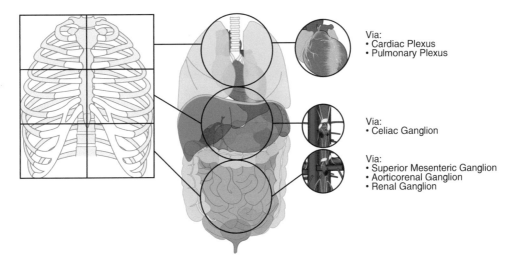

FIG. 33: A look at the organic influence of the ribs through the nervous system.

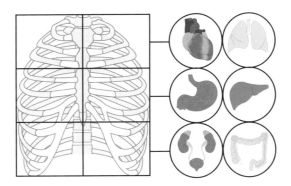

FIG. 34: Observing the rib divisions and the responsibility of the organs associated with each, we notice a pairing of organ functions. In the first division, we see heart and lung; in the second, stomach and liver; in the third, kidney and bladder and small and large intestines.

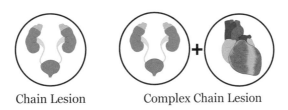

Chain Lesion   Complex Chain Lesion

FIG. 35: *Chain Lesion & Complex Chain Lesion.*

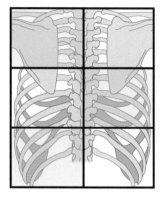

Example 1:
Unilateral Pattern
• Flexion upper left thorax
• Flexion middle right thorax
• Flexion lower left thorax

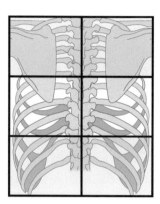

Example 2:
Bilateral Pattern
• Flexion upper thorax
• Extension middle thorax
• Flexion lower thorax

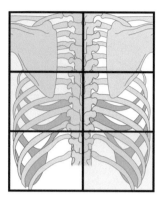

Example 3:
Other Patterns
• Flexion upper left thorax
• Flexion middle left thorax
• Flexion lower right thorax

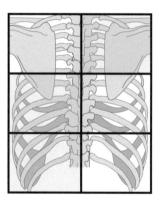

Example 4:
Other Patterns
• Flexion upper right thorax
• Flexion middle left thorax
• Flexion lower left thorax

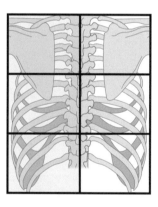

Example 5:
Other Patterns
• Flexion upper left thorax
• Flexion middle left thorax
• Flexion lower left thorax

FIG. 36: *Compensation within the six divisions.* Flexion is shown in blue.

3.2 Mechanics in Diagnosis and Treatment

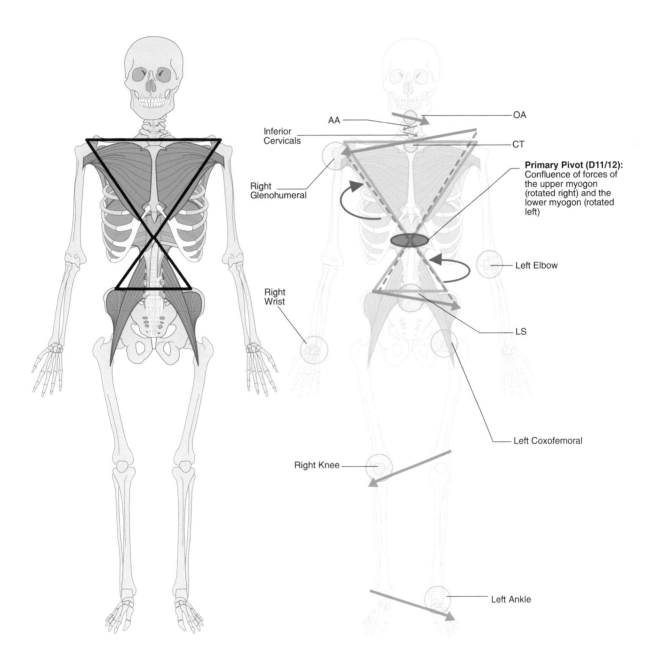

FIG. 37: *Theory of Compensation and Polygonal Mechanics.* Here we see Zink's Common Compensation Pattern overlaying polygonal mechanics in order to demonstrate the relationship between the two concepts.

Case Study #1

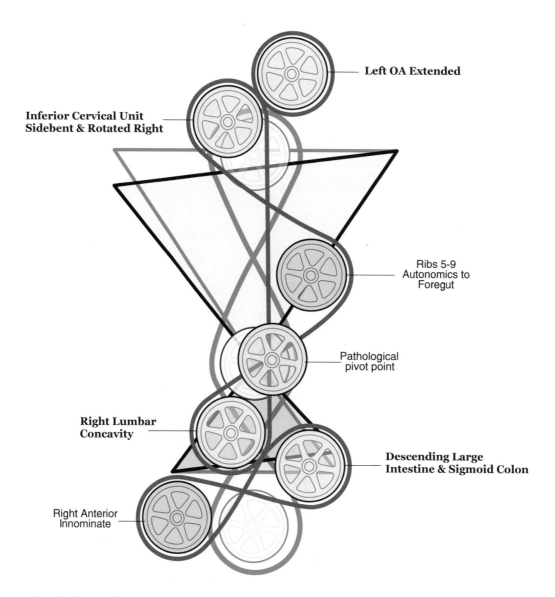

FIG. 38: *Case Study #1.*
• Patient presents with digestive complaints.
• Applying treatment to remove tension upon the descending colon results in more motion through the pelvis.
• Lesion of the left OA affects the vagus nerve and thus has major influence on the GI tract.
• Treatment of the inferior cervical unit (sidebent and rotated right) has a positive effect on motion of the OA joint.
• Lesioning at ribs 5-9 (which is related to the autonomics and to the digestive system). However, with correction of the right lumbar concavity, the rib lesion has softened.

Case Study #2

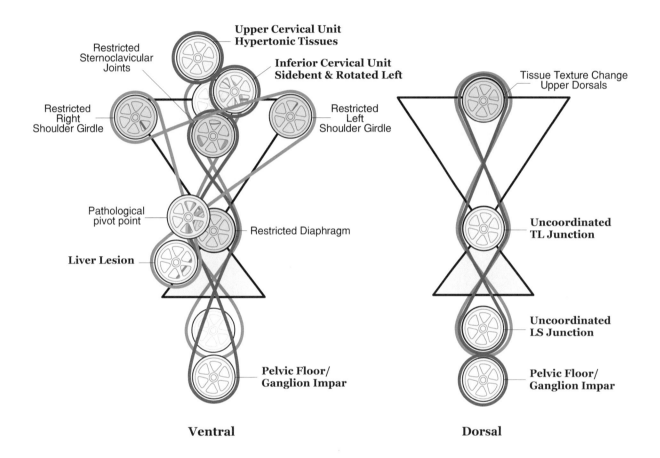

FIG. 39: *Case Study #2.*
• Patient presents as highly sympathetic and acute.
• Through the red belt we see the coordination of the nervous system in order to reduce the patient's sympathetic response. This is achieved mechanically through coordinating junctions, treatment of the pelvic floor, and upper and lower cervical units.
• Through the orange belt we see the connection between the tension around the liver, and the mobility of the shoulder girdles.

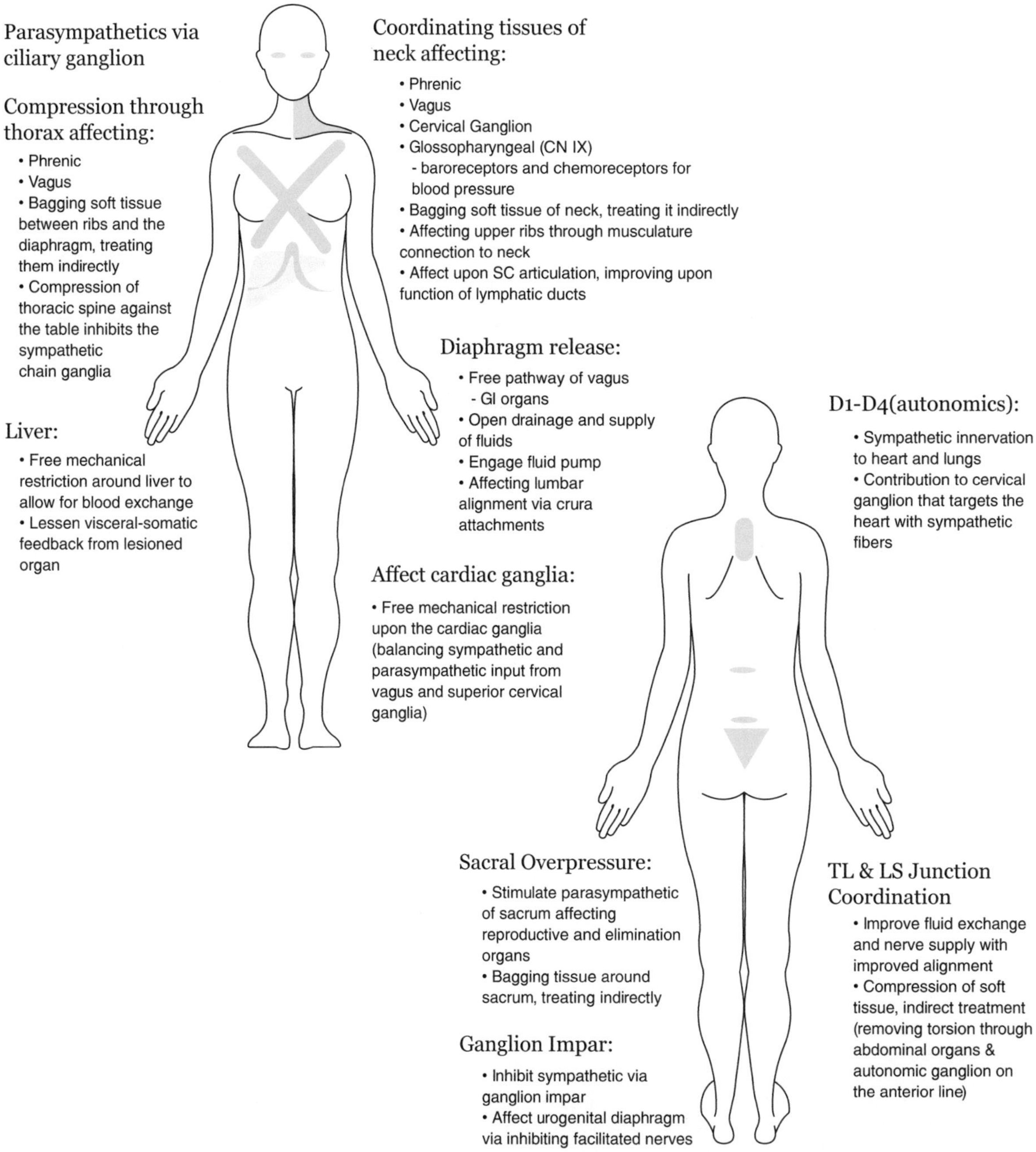

Parasympathetics via
ciliary ganglion

Compression through
thorax affecting:

• Phrenic
• Vagus
• Bagging soft tissue
between ribs and the
diaphragm, treating
them indirectly
• Compression of
thoracic spine against
the table inhibits the
sympathetic
chain ganglia

Liver:

• Free mechanical
restriction around liver to
allow for blood exchange
• Lessen visceral-somatic
feedback from lesioned
organ

Coordinating tissues of
neck affecting:

• Phrenic
• Vagus
• Cervical Ganglion
• Glossopharyngeal (CN IX)
  - baroreceptors and chemoreceptors for
  blood pressure
• Bagging soft tissue of neck, treating it indirectly
• Affecting upper ribs through musculature
connection to neck
• Affect upon SC articulation, improving upon
function of lymphatic ducts

Diaphragm release:

• Free pathway of vagus
  - GI organs
• Open drainage and supply
of fluids
• Engage fluid pump
• Affecting lumbar
alignment via crura
attachments

Affect cardiac ganglia:

• Free mechanical restriction
upon the cardiac ganglia
(balancing sympathetic and
parasympathetic input from
vagus and superior cervical
ganglia)

D1-D4(autonomics):

• Sympathetic innervation
to heart and lungs
• Contribution to cervical
ganglion that targets the
heart with sympathetic
fibers

Sacral Overpressure:

• Stimulate parasympathetic
of sacrum affecting
reproductive and elimination
organs
• Bagging tissue around
sacrum, treating indirectly

Ganglion Impar:

• Inhibit sympathetic via
ganglion impar
• Affect urogenital diaphragm
via inhibiting facilitated nerves

TL & LS Junction
Coordination

• Improve fluid exchange
and nerve supply with
improved alignment
• Compression of soft
tissue, indirect treatment
(removing torsion through
abdominal organs &
autonomic ganglion on
the anterior line)

FIG. 40: *Case Study #2. Neurophysiological Considerations.* Due to the nature of this case, the neurophysiological treatment considerations should be reflected upon.

Case Study #3

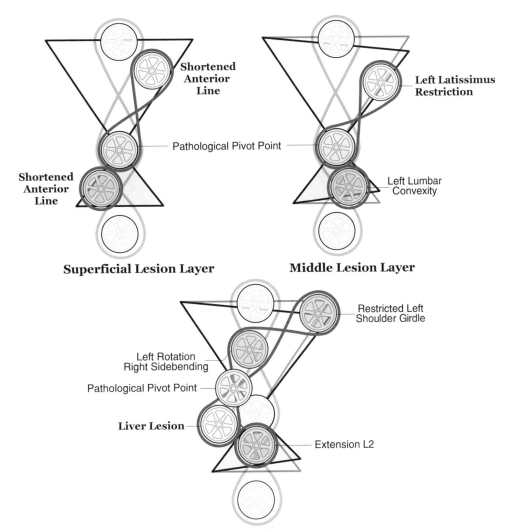

Superficial Lesion Layer

Middle Lesion Layer

Deepest Lesion Layer

FIG. 41: *Case Study #3.*
• Patient presents with a vascular urogenital dysfunction.

Superficial Lesion Layer (upper left): The upper and lower polygons are coordinated by removing the twist at the D/L junction.

Middle Lesion Layer (upper right): Restriction is noted through the lumbar concavity and is improved by working top down and treating the latissimus dorsi.

Deep Lesion Layer (right): Determining the primary lesion as the liver, treatment is applied, which results in an improvement of the STA and left shoulder.

Case Study #4

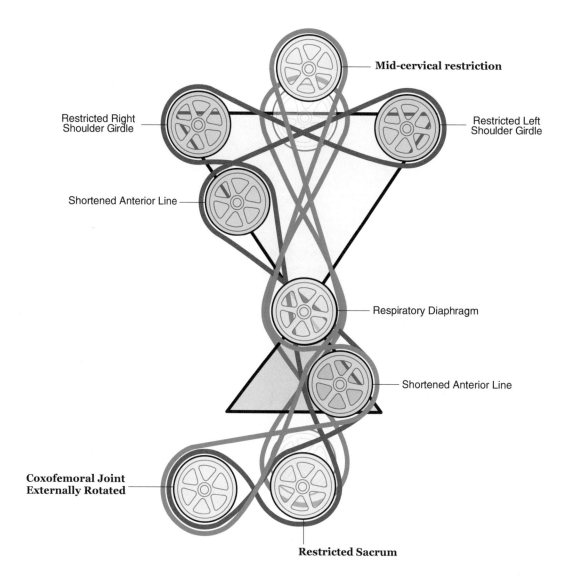

Mid-cervical restriction

Restricted Right
Shoulder Girdle

Restricted Left
Shoulder Girdle

Shortened Anterior Line

Respiratory Diaphragm

Shortened Anterior Line

Coxofemoral Joint
Externally Rotated

Restricted Sacrum

FIG. 42: *Case Study #4.*
• Patient presents with digestive issues.
• The red lesion belt demonstrates the resulting improvement found with correction of the sacral lesion, including improved should girdle motion and lessening of torsion through the abdominal field.
• The orange belt demonstrates the release of the lumbar spine and physiological changes at the epigastric fossa and respiratory diaphragm with correction of the cervical lesion.

Case Study #5

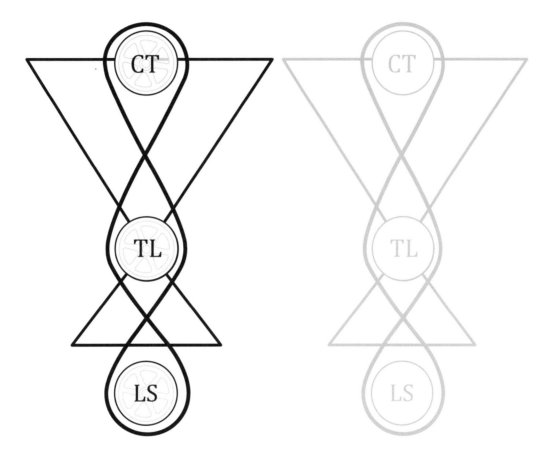

FIG. 43: *Case Study #5.*
These diagrams have been provided for the practitioner's use when applying the treatment algorithm described.

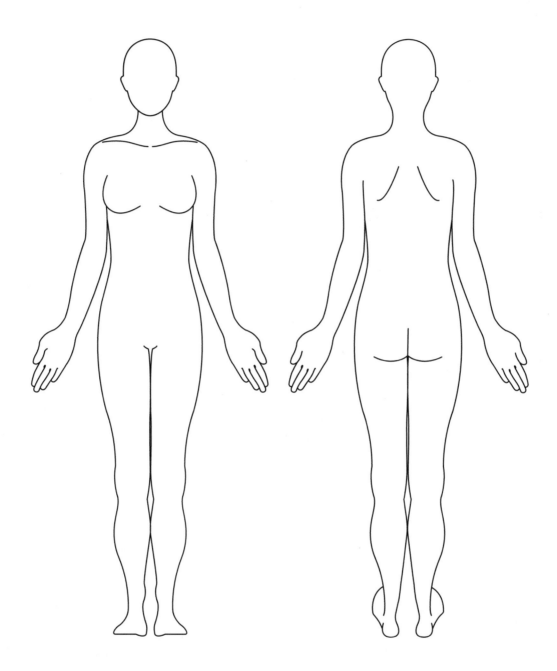

FIG. 43b

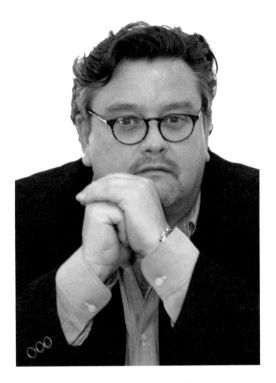

"I've always been passionate about instilling a new way of thinking in my classroom. Offering each student a unique learning experience tailored to their individual needs is a critical factor in establishing a successful educational program. Our course material isn't technique-driven or memorized from a textbook. It's designed to be hands-on, interactive, and really give students a legitimate understanding of human anatomy and physiology."

—Robert Johnston, CAO Principal

The faculty of the Canadian Academy of Osteopathy is headed by Robert Johnston. Mr. Johnston is Founder and Principal of the Canadian Academy of Osteopathy, and the Founder of both the Ontario Osteopathic Association, and the Canadian Institute of Classical Osteopathy. He is an enthusiastic and highly motivated clinical teacher and international lecturer who has dedicated his life to the promotion of Early American Classical Osteopathy. He has trained as a manual therapist in Canada, did his clinical internship in the United States, and trained directly under the late John Wernham in his post-graduate studies at the John Wernham College of Classical Osteopathy. Since then, it has been his goal to offer a progressive curriculum built on the proven theories and methodologies of Osteopathy's founding fathers. He continues to develop mechanical models for the student to approach osteopathic treatment. With ten years of experience as a clinical instructor and over twenty-five years of practice in manual therapy, Mr. Johnston possesses a rare talent for inspiring his students to reach the highest levels of academic performance.

Made in the USA
Columbia, SC
04 January 2025

51025115R00113